D1402370

Introduction to Healthcare

ATHENS TECHNICAL COLLEGE

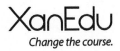

Copyright © 2014 by Athens Technical College.

All rights reserved

Printed in the United States of America

ISBN 13: 978-1-58390-131-1

No part of this book may be reprinted in any manner without written permission from the publisher.

Cover Images: Top: Copyright © Can Stock Photo, Inc./nmarques74; Bottom, left: Copyright © Can Stock Photo, Inc./Leaf; Bottom, center: Copyright © Copyright © Can Stock Photo, Inc./starman963; Bottom, right: Copyright © Can Stock Photo, Inc./creo77.

Acknowledgments:

pp. 2–23, 104–183: From *Diversified Health Occupations*, Seventh Edition, by Louise Simmers, Karen Simmers-Nartker, and Sharon Simmers-Kobelak. Copyright © 2009 by Delmar, Cengage Learning. Reprinted by permission of the publisher via the Copyright Clearance Center.

p. 25–73, 74–103: From *Diversified Health Occupations*, Sixth Edition, by Louise Simmers. Copyright © 2004 by Delmar, Cengage Learning. Reprinted by permission of the publisher via the Copyright Clearance Center.

p. 35: Figure 13-9 courtesy of and copyright © by Becton, Dickinson and Company. Reprinted by permission.

p. 36: Figure 13-10 "Standard Precautions" copyright © by Brevis Corporation. Reprinted by permission.

p. 66: Figure 13-42A, B copyright © Can Stock Photo, Inc./Lanesra.

p. 79: Figure 14-4 copyright © Omron Healthcare, Inc.

p. 129: Figure 16-19 copyright © by Ron Stram, MD.

pp. 147, 149: Figures 16-27A, 1627B, and 16-29 copyright © The Phoenix Society for Burn Survivors, Inc.

p. 152: Figure 16-31 copyright © Deborah Funk, MD.

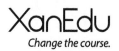

530 Great Road
Acton, MA 01720
800-562-2147

Contents

ALHS 1040
INTRODUCTION TO HEALTH CARE
MASTER COURSE SYLLABUS

Instructors will provide students with additional course-specific information, including attendance/makeup policies, assignment/test scheduling, and instructor contact information, as necessary and appropriate.

Prerequisite(s): Diploma program admission language competency or successful completion of required English and reading learning support courses with a grade of C* or higher

Co-requisite(s):	None
Term(s) Offered:	Every Semester
Class Hours:	2
Lab Hours:	3
Credit Hours:	3

Course Description

This course introduces a grouping of fundamental principles, practices, and issues common in the health care profession. In addition to the essential skills, students explore various delivery systems and related issues. Topics include basic life support/CPR, basic emergency care/first aid and triage, vital signs, infection control/blood and air-borne pathogens.

Course Competencies and Student Learning Outcomes

Infection control/blood and air-borne pathogens

Order	Description
1	Differentiate the roles, standards and guidelines for the following agencies: Center for Disease Control and Prevention (CDC); Occupational Health and Safety Administration (OSHA); and Federal Drug Administration (FDA).
2	Describe the characteristics of each link of the infection chain.
3	Define blood/air-borne pathogens.
4	Identify exposure risks related to health occupations.
5	Demonstrate pre and post exposure precautions to include handwashing, gloving (sterile/nonsterile, Personal Protective Equipment (PPE),
6	Describe causative agent, symptoms, occurrence, reservoir, mode of transmission, incubation period, period of communicability, prevention and control measures of the following diseases: Human Immunodeficiency Virus/Acquired Immunodeficiency Syndrome, all types of Hepatitis (A,B,C,), Tuberculosis, Meningitis, antibiotic resistant microbes and Herpes Viruses.
7	Differentiate forms of immunity.

Vital signs

Order	Description
1	Demonstrate proficiency in obtaining and documenting blood pressure, temperature, pulse,

respiration, weight and height.

2 Describe factors that affect vital signs including normal and abnormal values.

Basic emergency care/first aid and triage

Order	Description
1	A course from an accredited agency (American Safety and Health Institute, American Heart Association, American Red Cross) leading to certification in First Aid is acceptable in lieu of the following recommended outline.
2	Perform initial assessment.
3	Demonstrate various techniques for control of bleeding.
4	Describe first aid for various types of shock.
5	Apply bandages and splints.
6	Describe assessment and treatment of burns, poisoning, seizures, insect stings/bites, heat and cold exposure, syncope.

Basic life support/CPR

Order	Description
1	Acquire certification in CPR for Healthcare Providers (including 2 person CPR) by a certified instructor from American Heart Association or American Red Cross (or) CPR-PRO For the Professional Rescuer from the American Health and Safety Institute.

Required Textbook(s) and Materials

Students enrolled in this course are obligated to have the following:

Introduction to Healthcare, Technical College System of Georgia.

Basic Life Support (BLS) for Healthcare Providers Student Manual (90-1038). Current Edition

Grading Scale

The grading scale is detailed in the *Catalog and Student Handbook* and listed below for reference. All faculty members follow this scale when assigning grades to reflect a given student's performance in the classroom.

Grade	Numerical Equivalent	Grade Point
A/A*	90-100	4
B/B*	80-89	3
C/C*	70-79	2
D/D*	60-69	1
F/F*	0-59	0

Effective Summer Quarter 2006, Athens Technical College replaced the S/U grading system used for learning support classes with an A*-F* grading system. The registrar uses an asterisk (A*, B*, C*, D*, F*, W*, WF*, WP*) to designate learning support course grades on transcripts and grade reports because these grades are not components of the term grade point average.

Academic Support Center:

The Academic Support Centers of Athens Technical College (ATC) provide free tutoring for enrolled students. Both instructors and peer tutors provide tutoring in almost all subjects offered by the college. Information about the Center is accessible via the ATC website at http://www.athenstech.edu/StudentDevelopmentServices/AcademicSupportCenter. To find out the specific services available on the Athens, Greene, and Walton Campuses, please call (706) 583-2839. To contact the Academic Support Center on the Elbert County Campus, please call (706) 213-2129.

Attendance

Regular class attendance is important and expected. The college considers both tardiness and early departure from class as forms of absenteeism. Students absent from class for any reason are still responsible for all work missed. Instructors have the right to determine whether work missed can be made up and have the liberty to set reasonable expectations for attendance based on frequency of class meetings and on the instructional delivery method, subject, type, and level of the class. Class attendance policies will be clearly stated for students by their respective instructors on separate documents (course outlines/schedules) or appendices to the master syllabus.

Course Withdrawal

Students may withdraw from a course without academic penalty until the midpoint of the term. Students withdrawing after the midpoint of the term receive grades of WP – Withdrawal Passing, or WF – Withdrawal Failing. Students who stop attending class(es) without formally withdrawing risk earning a final grade of F, which will appear on the academic transcript. Withdrawing from a course may impact financial aid status, academic standing, and GPA. Refer to the ATC *Catalog and Student Handbook* for further details. http://www.athenstech.edu/Catalog/

Course Technology

Course addendum will provide details concerning the use of technology in the course. Course schedule types include **web-enhanced** – taught face-to-face; **online** – taught online using the internet, may require proctored exam; **hybrid** – class time is split between face-to-face and online; **video conference** – taught at two or more campus locations simultaneously with instructor located at one of the classroom locations. More details are available on the Athens Technical College website. http://www.athenstech.edu/eLearning/CourseList.cfm

Continuation of Instruction

In the event of severe weather or other emergency, students will be expected to continue participating in learning activities via ANGEL, Athens Technical College email, or other modality. Instructors will provide a plan for the continuation of instruction.

Work Ethics:

To fulfill the responsibility to teach essential workplace ethics, the college provides students instruction in, and evaluates students on, the following ten work ethics traits: attendance, character, teamwork, appearance, attitude, productivity, organizational skills, communication, cooperation, and respect. To best equip students for successful workplace experiences in their chosen profession, instruction and evaluation takes place in the context of their program of study.

Academic Honesty

Academic honesty is expected at all times. Any student found to have engaged in academic misconduct such as cheating, plagiarism, or collusion is subject to disciplinary sanctions as outlined in the Student Code of Conduct detailed in the ATC *Catalog and Student Handbook* . See the following link for the complete Academic Honesty policy. http://www.athenstech.edu/StudentAffairs/AcademicHonesty/Academic%20Honesty.pdf
Students are also advised to complete the tutorial on Academic Honesty available here: http://www/athenstech.edu/StudentAffairs/AcademicHonesty

Americans with Disabilities Act

It is our goal at Athens Technical College to provide equal access to education for all students. Any student with a documented disability is eligible to receive reasonable academic adjustments and auxiliary aids in the classroom and/or for testing at Athens Technical College, as long as appropriate documentation of the disability has been submitted to the Disability Services Office in a timely manner. Students can access the application packet on our website. http://www.athenstech.edu/CurrentStudents/orientation/files/disability_services_application.pdf

Cell Phones and Electronic Devices

Cell phone use in the classroom for non-instructional purposes, with the exception of receiving emergency notifications, is prohibited.

Food/Drinks in Classroom

Food and beverages (other than water) are not allowed in classrooms/labs.

Communication with ATC Faculty and Staff

Students, faculty, and staff must use Athens Technical College email and ANGEL accounts for all college-related communications. Students are obligated to check their email and ANGEL accounts on a regular basis, preferably daily.

Warranty of Graduates

The Technical College System of Georgia warranties every graduate of technical programs in which students may earn technical certificates of credit, diplomas, or associate degrees. The warranty guarantees that graduates demonstrate the knowledge and skills and can perform each competency as identified in the industry-validated standards established for every program of study. If one of our graduates educated under a standard program or his/her employer finds that the graduate is deficient in one or more competencies as defined in the course/program standards, Athens Technical College will retrain the employee at no instructional cost to the employee or the employer. This guarantee is in effect for two years after graduation.

TEACH Act

According to the TEACH Act of 2002, Athens Technical College is obligated to advise you that instructional material included in this course may be subject to copyright protection. As such, you must not share, duplicate, transmit, or store the material of this course beyond the purpose and time frame explicitly stated in the syllabus of your course. If you are not certain whether a particular piece of material is covered by copyright protection, you should contact your instructor and obtain his/her written clarification. Failing to observe copyright protection is a violation of law.

CHAPTER 1

Preparing for the World of Work

Chapter Objectives

After completing this chapter,
you should be able to:

- Identify at least five job-keeping skills and explain why employers consider them to be essential skills

- Write a cover letter containing all required information and using correct form for letters

- Prepare a résumé containing all necessary information and meeting standards for neatness and correctness

- Complete a job application form that meets standards of neatness and accuracy

- Demonstrate how to participate in a job interview, including wearing correct dress and meeting standards established in this chapter

- Determine gross and net income

- Calculate an accurate budget for a one-month period, accounting for fixed expenses and variable expenses without exceeding net monthly income

- Define, pronounce, and spell all key terms

Observe Standard Precautions

Instructor's Check—Call Instructor at This Point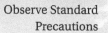

Safety—Proceed with Caution

OBRA Requirement—Based on Federal Law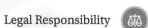

Math Skill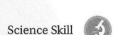

Legal Responsibility

Science Skill

Career Information

Communications Skill

Technology

KEY TERMS

application forms	fixed expenses	letter of application
budget	gross income	net income
cover letter	income	résumé *(rez'-ah-may)*
deductions	job interview	variable expenses

17:1 INFORMATION

Developing Job-Keeping Skills

To obtain and keep a job you must develop certain characteristics to be a good employee. A recent survey of employers asked for information on the deficiencies of high school graduates. The most frequent complaints included poor written grammar, spelling, speech, and math skills. Other complaints included lack of respect for work, lack of self-initiative, poor personal appearance, not accepting responsibility, excessive tardiness, poor attendance, and inability to accept criticism. Any of these defects would be detrimental in a health care worker.

It is essential that you develop good job-keeping skills to be successful in a health care career. Being aware of and striving to achieve the qualities needed for employment are as important as acquiring the knowledge and skills required in your chosen health care profession.

Job-keeping skills include:

◆ *Use correct grammar at all times.* This includes both the written and spoken word. Patients often judge ability on how well a person speaks or writes information. Use of words like *ain't* indicates a lack of education and does not create a favorable or professional impression. You must constantly strive to use correct grammar. Listen to how other health care professionals speak and review basic concepts of correct grammar. It may even be necessary to take a communications course to learn to speak correctly. Because you will be completing legal written records for health care, the use of correct spelling, punctuation, and sentence structure is also essential. Use a dictionary to check spelling, or use the spell check on a computer system. Refer to standard English books or secretarial manuals for information on sentence structure and punctuation. Constantly strive to improve both oral and written communication skills.

◆ *Report to work on time and when scheduled.* Because many health care facilities provide care 7 days a week, 365 days per year, and often 24 hours per day, an employee who is frequently late or absent can cause a major disruption in schedule and contribute to an insufficiency of personnel to provide patient care. Most health care facilities have strict rules regarding absenteeism, and a series of absences can result in job loss.

◆ *Be prepared to work when you arrive at work.* An employer does not pay workers to socialize, make personal telephone calls, consult others about personal or family problems, bring their children to work, shop on the Internet, play games on a computer, or work in a sloppy and inefficient manner. Develop a good work ethic. Observe all legal and ethical responsibilities. Follow the policies and procedures of your health care facility. Recognize your limitations and seek help when you need it. Be willing to learn new procedures and techniques. Watch efficient and knowledgeable staff members and learn by their examples. Constantly strive to do the best job possible. A worker who has self-initiative, who sees a job that needs to be done and does it, is a valuable employee who is likely to be recognized and rewarded.

◆ *Practice teamwork.* Because health care typically involves a team of different professionals working together to provide patient care, it is important to be willing to work with others. If you are willing to help others when they need help, they will likely be willing to help you. Two or three people working together can lift a heavy patient much more readily than can one.

♦ *Promote a positive attitude.* By being positive, you create a good impression and encourage the same attitude in others. Too often, employees concentrate only on the negative aspects of their jobs. Every job has some bad points; and it is easy to criticize these points. It is also easy to criticize the bad points in others with whom you work. However, this leads to a negative attitude and helps create poor morale in everyone. By concentrating on the good aspects of a job and the rewards it can provide, work will seem much more pleasant, and employees will obtain more satisfaction from their efforts.

♦ *Accept responsibility for your actions.* Most individuals are more than willing to take credit for the good things they have done. In the same manner, it is essential to take responsibility for mistakes. If you make a mistake, report it to your supervisor and make every effort to correct the error. Every human being will do something wrong at some time. Recognizing an error, taking responsibility for it, and making every effort to correct it or prevent it from happening again is a sign of a competent worker. Honesty is essential in health care. Not accepting responsibility for your actions is dishonest. It is often a reason for dismissal and can prevent you from obtaining another position.

♦ *Be willing to learn.* Health care changes constantly because of advances in technology and research. Every health care worker must be willing to learn new things and adapt to change. Participating in staff development programs (figure 17-1), taking courses at technical schools or colleges, attending special seminars or meetings, reading professional journals, and asking questions of other qualified individuals are all ways to improve your knowledge and skills. Employers recognize these efforts. Ambition is often rewarded with a higher salary and/or job advancement.

Without good job-keeping skills, no amount of knowledge will help you keep a job. Therefore, it is essential for you to strive to develop the qualities that employers need in workers. Be courteous, responsible, enthusiastic, cooperative, reliable, punctual, and efficient. Strive hard

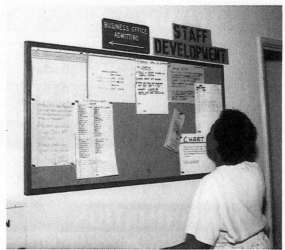

FIGURE 17-1 Participating in staff development programs is one way to improve your own knowledge and skills.

to be the best you can be. If you do this, you will not only be likely to retain your job, but you will probably be rewarded with job advancement, increased salary, and personal satisfaction.

STUDENT: *Go to the workbook and complete the assignment sheet for 17:1, Developing Job-Keeping Skills.*

17:2 INFORMATION

Writing a Cover Letter and Preparing a Résumé

INTRODUCTION

Before you look for a job, evaluate your interests and abilities. Decide what type job you would like. Make sure you obtain the education needed to perform the job. Then look at different job sources to try to find a position you will like. There are many different sources for finding job openings. Some of them include:

♦ Advertisements in newspapers

♦ Job fairs sponsored by schools or employment agencies

♦ Recommendations from friends and relatives

♦ School counselors or bulletin boards

♦ Employment agencies

- Internet job search sites
- Professional organizations: check their Internet site or contact the local organization
- Job listings posted at health care facilities or listed on their Internet site

Once you have identified possible places of employment, prepare to apply for the position. In most cases, this involves writing a cover letter, or letter of application, and a résumé.

COVER LETTER

The purpose of a **cover letter** or **letter of application** is to obtain an interview. You must create a good impression in the letter so that the employer will be interested in hiring you. In many cases, you will be responding to a job advertised either in the newspaper, on the Internet, or through other sources. However a résumé may be sent to potential employers even though they have not advertised a job opportunity. A cover letter should accompany all résumés.

The letter should be computer printed or typewritten on good quality paper. It must be neat, complete, and done according to correct form for letters. The correct form for composing business letters is discussed in detail in Chapter 23:5 of this textbook. Care must be taken to ensure that spelling and punctuation are correct. Remember, this letter is the employer's first impression of you.

If possible, the letter should be addressed to the correct individual. If you know the name of the agency or company, call to obtain this information. Be sure you obtain the correct spelling of the person's name as well as the person's correct title. If you are responding to a box number, follow the instructions in the advertisement. Another possibility is to address the letter to the director of human resources or the head of a particular department.

The letter usually contains three to four paragraphs. The contents of each paragraph are described as follows:

- *Paragraph one*: state your purpose for writing and express interest in the position for which you are applying. If you are responding to an advertisement, state the name and date of the publication. If you were referred by another individual, give this person's name and title.

- *Paragraph two*: state why you believe you are qualified for the position. It may also state why you want to work for this particular employer. Information should be brief because most of the information will be included on your résumé.

- *Paragraph three*: state that a résumé is included. You may also want to draw the employer's attention to one or two important features on your résumé. If you are not including a résumé, state that one is available on request. Whenever possible, it is best to enclose a résumé.

- *Paragraph four*: closes the letter with a request for an interview. Be sure you clearly state how the employer can contact you for additional information. Include a telephone number and the times you will be available to respond to a telephone call. Finally, include a thank you to the potential employer for considering your application.

Figure 17-2 is a sample cover letter to serve as a guide to writing a good letter. However, remember this is only one guide. Letters must be varied to suit each circumstance.

RÉSUMÉ

A **résumé** is a record of information about an individual. It is a thorough yet concise summary of an individual's education, skills, accomplishments, and work experience. It is used to provide an employer with basic information that makes you appear qualified as an employee. At the same time, a good résumé will help you clarify your job objective and be better prepared for a job interview.

A résumé should be computer printed or typed and attractive in appearance. Like a cover letter, a résumé creates an impression on the employer. Information should be presented in an organized fashion. At the same time, the résumé should be concise and pertinent. Good-quality paper; correct spelling and punctuation; straight, even margins; and an attractive style are essential. If an individual is sending out a series of résumés, professional copies are permitted. However, the copies must be clear, on good-quality paper, and appealing in appearance.

Résumé format can vary. Review sample sources and find a style that you feel best pre-

```
18 Hireme Lane
Job City, Ohio 44444
June 3, 20--


Mr. Prospective Employer
Director of Human Resources
Health Care Facility
12 Nursing Lane
Dental City, Ohio 44833

Dear Mr. Employer:

In response to your advertisement in the _____
on _____, 20 _____, I would like to apply for
the position of _____.

I recently graduated from _____. I majored in
_____ and feel I am well qualified for this
position. I enjoy working with people and have a sincere
interest in additional training in _____.

My resume is enclosed. I have also enclosed a specific list of
skills that I mastered during my school experience. I feel
that previous positions noted on the resume have provided me
with a good basis for meeting your job requirements.

Thank you for considering my application. I would appreciate
a personal interview at your earliest convenience to discuss
my qualifications. Please contact me at the above address or
by telephone at 589-1111 after 2:00 PM any day.


Sincerely,


Iamjob Hunting
```

FIGURE 17-2 A sample cover letter.

sents your information. A one-page résumé is usually sufficient.

Parts of a résumé can also vary. Some of the most important parts that should be included are shown in figures 17-3A and 17-3B and are described as follows:

♦ *Personal identification*: This includes your name, address, and telephone number. Be sure to include the area code.

♦ *Employment objective, job desired, or career goal*: Briefly state the title of the position for which you are applying.

Florence Nurse
22 South Main Street
Nursing, Ohio 33303
(400)589-1111

Employment Objective: Nursing Assistant Position

Skills

Recording Vital Signs	Making Beds
Moving and Transferring Patients	Observing Infection Control
Administrering CPR and First Aid	Providing Personal Hygience
Understanding Medical Terminology	Collecting Specimens
Applying Heat or Cold Applications	Ambulating Patients

Education

Career High School	Graduation: June 5, 2008
5 Diamond Street	Major: Health Occupations
Nursing, Ohio 33303	Grade Average: A's and B's

Certification: State Approved Nurse Assistant

Work Experience

Summer 2007 to Present	Country King Fried Chicken
	5 Southern Lane
	Mansfield, Ohio 33302
Fast Food Worker	Operate register
	Record orders
	Promote customer relations
Summer of 2005 and 2008	Madison Ram Hospital
	602 Esley Lane
	Mansfield, Ohio 33301
Volunteer Worker	Deliver mail and flowers
	Assist nurses with patients

Extracurricular Activities

School Marching Band	Member for 3 years
SkillsUSA	Class treasurer for 2 years
Red Cross Club	Member for 3 years
Red Cross Blood Mobile	Volunteer worker for 3 years
March of Dimes Walkathon	Walker for 5 years
Church Youth Group	Member for 7 years

FIGURE 17-3A A sample résumé with information centered.

THOMAS J. TOOTH

| 340 DENTAL LANE | FLOSS, OHIO 44598 | (524) 333-2435 |

CAREER GOAL: POSITION AS A DENTAL ASSISTANT IN GENERAL PRACTICE WITH A GOAL OF BECOMING A CERTIFIED DENTAL ASSISTANT

EDUCATION: OHIO JOINT VOCATIONAL SCHOOL, OPPORTUNITY, OHIO 44597
GRADUATED IN JUNE 2007
MAJORED IN DENTAL ASSISTANT PROGRAM FOR TWO YEARS

SKILLS: IDENTIFICATION OF TEETH, CHARTING CONDITIONS OF THE TEETH, MIXING DENTAL CEMENTS AND BASES, POURING MODELS AND CUSTOM TRAYS, PREPARING ANESTHETIC SYRINGE, SETTING UP BASIC DENTAL TRAYS, STERILIZING OF INSTRUMENTS, DEVELOPING AND MOUNTING RADIOGRAPHS, TYPING BUSINESS LETTERS, COMPLETING INSURANCE FORMS

WORK EXPERIENCE: DENTAL LAB PRODUCTS, 55 MODEL STREET, FLOSS, OHIO 44598
EMPLOYED SEPTEMBER 2006 TO PRESENT AS DENTAL LAB ASSISTANT
PROFICIENT IN MODELS, CUSTOM TRAYS, PROSTHETIC DEVICES

DRUGGIST STORES, 890 PHARMACY LANE, OPPORTUNITY, OHIO 44597
EMPLOYED JUNE 2004 TO AUGUST 2006 AS SALESPERSON
EXPERIENCE IN CUSTOMER RELATIONS, INVENTORY, REGISTER, AND SALES PROMOTION

ACTIVITIES: HEALTH OCCUPATIONS STUDENTS OF AMERICA (HOSA) TREASURER
FIRST PLACE STATE AWARD IN HOSA DENTAL ASSISTANT CONTEST
VOLUNTEER WORKER DURING DENTAL HEALTH WEEK
MEMBER OF SCHOOL PEP CLUB
HOBBIES INCLUDE FOOTBALL, SWIMMING, BASKETBALL, READING
VOLUNTEER FOR MEALS-ON-WHEELS

PERSONAL TRAITS: DEPENDABLE, CONSIDERATE OF OTHERS, WILLING TO LEARN, ADAPTABLE TO NEW SITUATIONS, RESPECTFUL AND HONEST, ADEPT AT DENTAL TERMINOLOGY, ABLE TO PERFORM A VARIETY OF DENTAL SKILLS

FIGURE 17-3B A sample résumé with left margin highlights.

◆ *Educational background*: List the name and address of your high school. Be sure to include special courses or majors if they relate to the job position. If you have taken additional courses or special training, list them also. If you have completed college or technical school, this information should be placed first.

◆ *Work or employment experience*: This includes previous positions of employment. Always start with the most recent position and work backward. Each entry should include the name and address of the employer, dates employed, your job title, and a brief description of duties. Avoid use of the word *I*. For example, instead of stating, "I sterilized supplies," state, "sterilized supplies," using action verbs to describe duties.

◆ *Skills*: List special knowledge, computer, and work skills you have that can be used in the job you are seeking. The list of skills should be specific and indicate your qualifications and ability to perform the job duties. When work experience is limited, a list of skills is important to show an employer that you are qualified for the position.

◆ *Other activities*: These can include organizations of which you are a member, offices held, community activities, special awards received, volunteer work, hobbies, special interests, and other similar facts. Keep this information brief, but do not hesitate to include facts that indicate school, church, and community involvement. This section can show an employer that you are a well-rounded person who participates in activities, assumes leadership roles, strives to achieve, and practices good citizenship. Write out the full names of organizations rather than the identifying letters.

◆ *References*: Most sources recommend not including references on a resume. Even the statement "references will be furnished on request" is now usually omitted. However, at least three references should be placed on a separate sheet of paper. The paper should be the same paper used for the résumé and include the same heading showing your name, address, and telephone number. The reference sheet can be given to an employer during the job interview. For a high school student with limited experience, references can provide valuable additional information. Always be sure you have an individual's permission before using that person as a reference. List the full name, title, address, and telephone number of the reference. It is best not to use relatives or high school friends as references. Select professionals in your field, clergy, teachers, or other individuals with responsible positions.

Honesty is always the best policy, and this is particularly true regarding résumés. Never give information that you think will look good but is exaggerated or only partly true. Inaccurate or false information can cost you a job. If you have an A to B average in school, include this information. If your average is lower than an A to B, do *not* include this information.

Before preparing your résumé, it is important to list all of the information you wish to include. Then select the format that best presents this information. The two sample résumés shown in figures 17-3A and 17-3B are meant to serve as guidelines only. Do not hesitate to evaluate other formats and present your information in the best possible way.

The envelope should be the correct size for your letter of application and résumé. Do *not* fold the letter into small sections and put it in an undersized envelope. This creates a sloppy impression. When possible, it is best to buy standard business envelopes that match your paper. A 9 × 12 envelope eliminates the need to fold the cover letter and résumé, and helps create a more professional appearance. Be sure the envelope is addressed correctly and neatly. It should also be computer printed or typewritten.

CAREER PASSPORT OR PORTFOLIO

A *career passport* or *portfolio* is a professional way to highlight your knowledge, abilities, and skills as you prepare for employment or extended education. It allows you to present yourself in an organized and efficient manner when you interview for schools or employment. Most career passports or portfolios contain the following types of information:

◆ *Introductory letter*: provides a brief synopsis of yourself including your background, education, and future goals

◆ *Résumé*: provides an organized record of information on education, employment experience, special skills, and activities

◆ *Skill list and competency level*: provides a list of skills you have mastered and the level of competency for each skill; some health occupation programs provide summaries of competency evaluations that can be used; if your program does not provide this, a list of skills and final competency grades can be compiled by using the evaluation sheets in the *Diversified Health Occupations Workbook*

◆ *Letter(s) of recommendation*: include letters of recommendation from your instructors, guidance counselors, supervisors at clinical areas or agencies where you perform volunteer work, respected members of the community, advisors of activities in which you participate, and presidents of organizations of which you are a member

◆ *Copies of work evaluations*: include copies of evaluations you receive at job-training sites, volunteer activities, and/or paid work experiences

◆ *Documentation of mastering job-keeping skills*: the federal government has created SCANS, or the Secretaries Commission on Acquiring Necessary Skills, to designate skills employers desire in employees. SCANS lists three foundation skills that employers desire: *basic skills* (able to read, write, solve math problems, speak, and listen), *thinking skills* (able to learn, reason, think creatively, make decisions, and solve problems), and *personal qualities* (display responsibility, self-initiative, sociability, honesty, and integrity). In addition, SCANS lists five workplace competencies: *manage resources* (demonstrate ability to allocate time, money, materials, and space), *display interpersonal skills* (demonstrate ability to work in a team, lead, negotiate, compromise, teach others, and work with individuals from diverse backgrounds), *utilize information* (acquire and evaluate data, file information, interpret information, and communicate with others), *comprehend systems* (understand social, organizational, and technical systems), and *use technologies* (use computers, apply technology to specific tasks, and maintain equipment). Write brief paragraphs to document how you have mastered skills such as teamwork, self-motivation, leadership, a willingness to learn, responsibility, organization, and other SCANS qualities

◆ *Leadership and organization abilities*: include information that demonstrates leadership and organization abilities you have mastered; participation in HOSA or Skills USA should be included

Organize the above information in a neat binder or portfolio. Use tab dividers to separate it into organized sections. Make sure that you use correct grammar and punctuation on all written information. The effort you put into creating a professional portfolio or passport will be beneficial when you have this document ready to present during a school or job interview.

STUDENT: *Go to the workbook and complete the assignment sheet for 17:2, Writing a Cover Letter and Résumé. Then return and continue with the procedure.*

PROCEDURE 17:2

Writing a Cover Letter and Preparing a Résumé

Equipment and Supplies

Good-quality paper, inventory sheet for résumés (see workbook), computer with word processing software and a printer, or typewriter

Procedure

1. Assemble equipment.

2. Re-read the preceding information section on a cover letter and résumés. Read the section on Composing Business Letters in Chapter 23:5 of this textbook.

3. Review the sample letters of application and résumés.

4. Go to the workbook and complete the inventory sheet for résumés. Check dates for accuracy. Be sure that names are spelled correctly. Use the telephone book or other sources to check addresses and zip codes.

5. Carefully evaluate all your information. Determine the best method of present-

PROCEDURE 17:2

ing your information. Try different ways of writing your material. Do not hesitate to show several different versions to your instructor or others and get their opinions on which way seems most effective.

6. Type a rough draft of a cover letter. Follow the correct form for letters as shown in Chapter 23:5 of this textbook. Use correct spacing and margins. Check for correct spelling and punctuation.

7. Type a final cover letter. Be sure it contains the required information. Proofread the letter for spelling errors and other mistakes. If possible, ask someone else to proofread your letter and evaluate it.

8. Type a rough draft of your résumé. Position the information in an attractive manner. Be sure that spacing is standard throughout the résumé and margins are even on all sides.

9. Review your sample résumé. Reword any information, if necessary. Be sure all information is pertinent and concise. Ask your instructor or others for opinions regarding suggested changes.

10. Type your final résumé. Take care to avoid errors. If you are not a good typist, it might be wise to have someone else complete the final draft. Proofread the

final copy, checking carefully for errors. If possible, ask someone else to proofread your résumé and evaluate it.

NOTE: Résumés can be copies of the original; but be sure the copies are of good quality. Cover letters must be originals; they are individually tailored for each potential job, and, therefore, are not copied.

11. Replace all equipment.

Practice

Go to the workbook and use the evaluation sheet for 17:2, Writing a Cover Letter and Résumé, to practice this procedure. When you believe you have mastered this skill, sign the sheet and give it to your instructor for further action. Also give your instructor your cover letter and résumé along with the evaluation sheet.

 Final Checkpoint Using the criteria listed on the evaluation sheet, your instructor will grade your cover letter and résumé.

17:3 INFORMATION

Completing Job Application Forms

Even though you provide each potential employer with a résumé, most employers still require you to complete an application form. **Application forms** are used by employers to collect specific information. Forms vary from employer to employer, but most request similar information.

Before completing any application form, it is essential that you first read the entire form. Note

areas where certain information is to be placed. Read instructions that state how the form is to be completed. Some forms request that the applicant type or print all answers. Others request that the form be completed in the person's handwriting. If a scanner is available, an application form can be scanned into a computer so information can be keyed onto the application. The application can then be printed. Some health care facilities are using online applications. A computer is used to key information into the appropriate spaces. The application form is then printed and mailed or sent electronically by e-mail to the employer.

Be sure you have all the required information with you when you go for a job interview. Many employers will ask you to complete the application form at that time. Others will allow you to take the form home. Still others will even send the form to you prior to the interview. The latter two options allow you more time to obtain complete information and print or type the form (unless otherwise requested).

Basic rules for completing a job application form include:

♦ Fill out each item neatly and completely.

♦ Do *not* leave any areas blank. Put "none" or "NA" (meaning "not applicable") when the item requested does not apply to you.

♦ Be sure addresses include zip codes and all other required information.

♦ Watch spelling and punctuation. Errors will not impress the potential employer.

♦ Type or print neatly if the application does not state otherwise.

♦ Use a black pen if printing.

♦ If possible, scan the application into a computer word program, key in all information, check for accuracy, and then print the completed application form. Use spell-check if it is available. This method allows for easy correction of errors.

♦ Make sure all information is legible.

♦ Do *not* write in spaces that state "office use only" or "do not write below this line." Employers often judge how well you follow directions by your reaction to these sections.

♦ Be sure all information is correct and truthful. Remember, material can be checked and verified. A simple half-truth can cost you a job.

♦ Proofread your completed application. Check for completeness, spelling, proper answers to questions, and any errors.

♦ If references are requested, be sure to include all information such as title, address, and telephone number. Before using anyone's name as a reference, it is best to obtain that person's permission. Be prepared to provide reference information when you go for a job interview. Most sources suggest listing at least three references on a separate sheet of the same type of paper used for the résumé.

Even though questions vary on different forms, some basic information is usually requested on all of them. In order to be sure you have this information, it is useful to take a "wallet card" with you. A sample card is included in the workbook (as Assignment 2). Employers will not be impressed if you have to ask for a telephone book to find requested information; you may appear to be unprepared. Of course, if you are allowed to take the application home or if it is mailed or sent electronically (e-mail) to you, looking for information would not be a problem.

Remember that employers use application forms as a screening method. To avoid being eliminated from consideration for a position of employment, be sure your application creates a favorable impression.

STUDENT: *Go to the workbook and complete the assignment sheets for 17:3, Completing Job Application Forms and Wallet Card. Then return and continue with the procedure.*

PROCEDURE 17:3

Completing Job Application Forms

Equipment and Supplies

Typewriter or computer and scanner or pen, wallet card (sample in workbook), sample application forms (sample in workbook)

Procedure

1. Assemble equipment. If a typewriter is used, be sure the ribbon is of good quality. If a scanner is available, scan the application form into the word processing program of a computer. The application form can then be completed with the computer and printed on a printer.

PROCEDURE 17:3

2. Complete all information on the wallet card. A sample is included in the workbook (as Assignment 2). Check dates and be sure information is accurate. List full addresses, zip codes, and names.

3. Review the preceding information section on completing job application forms. Read additional references, as needed.

4. Read the entire sample application form (Assignment 3) in the workbook. Be sure you understand the information requested for each part. Read all directions completely.

5. Unless otherwise directed, type all information requested. If a typewriter is not available, use a black ink pen to print all information. If a scanner and computer are available, scan the application form into a word program. After keying in all information, the completed application can be printed.

6. Complete all areas of the form. Use "none" or "NA" as a reply to items that do not apply to you.

7. Take care not to write in spaces labeled "office use only" or "do not write below this line." Leave these areas blank.

8. In the space labeled "signature," sign your name. Note any statement that may be printed by the signature line. Be sure you are aware of what you are signing and the permission you may be giving. Most employers request permission to contact previous employers and/or references, and a verification that information is accurate.

9. Recheck the entire application. Be sure information is correct and complete. Note and correct any spelling errors. Be sure you have answered all of the questions.

10. Replace all equipment.

Practice

Go to the workbook and use the evaluation sheet for 17:3, Completing Job Application Forms, to practice this procedure. Obtain sample job application forms from your instructor or other sources. When you believe you have mastered this skill, sign the sheet and give it to your instructor for further action.

 Final Checkpoint Using the criteria listed on the evaluation sheet, your instructor will grade your job application form.

17:4 INFORMATION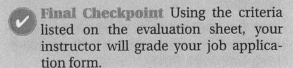

Participating in a Job Interview

A job interview is what you are seeking when you send a letter of application and a résumé. You must prepare for an interview just as hard as you did when composing your résumé. A poor interview can mean a lost job.

A **job interview** is usually the last step before getting or being denied a particular position of employment. Usually, you have been screened by the potential employer and have been selected for an interview as a result of your résumé and application form. To the employer, the interview serves at least two main purposes:

◆ Provides the opportunity to evaluate you in person, obtain additional information, and ascertain whether you meet the job qualifications

◆ Allows the employer to tell you about the position in more detail

Careful preparation is needed before going to an interview. Be sure you have all required information. Your "wallet card," résumé, and completed application form (if you have done one) must be ready. If you have completed a career passport or portfolio, be sure to take it to the interview. If possible, find out about the position and the agency offering the job. In this way, you will be more aware of the agency's needs.

Be sure of the scheduled date and time of the interview. Know the name of the individual you must contact and the exact place of the interview. Write this information down and take it with you.

Dress carefully. It is best to dress conservatively. Coats and ties are still best for men. Although pantsuits are sometimes acceptable for women, employers still generally prefer dresses or skirts. Even though it shouldn't be the case, first impressions can affect the employer. All clothes should fit well and be clean and pressed, if needed. Avoid bright, flashy colors and very faddish styles.

Check your entire appearance. Hair should be neat, clean, and styled attractively. Nails should be clean. Women should avoid wearing bright nail polish, too much makeup, and perfume. Men should be clean shaven. Be sure that your teeth are clean and your breath is fresh. Jewelry should not be excessive. And last but not least, use a good antiperspirant. When you are nervous, you perspire.

It is best to arrive 5–10 minutes early for your interview. Late arrival could mean a lost job. Allow for traffic, trains blocking the road, and other complications that might interfere with your arriving on time.

During the interview, observe all of the following points:

♦ Greet the interviewer by name when you are introduced. Introduce yourself. Shake hands firmly and smile (figure 17-4A).

♦ Remain standing until the interviewer asks you to sit. Be aware of your posture and sit straight. Keep both feet flat on the floor or cross your legs at the ankles only.

♦ Use correct grammar. Avoid using slang words.

♦ Speak slowly and clearly. Don't mumble.

♦ Be polite. Practice good manners.

♦ Maintain eye contact (figure 17-4B). Avoid looking at the floor, ceiling, or away from the interviewer. Looking at the middle of the interviewer's forehead or at the tip of the interviewer's nose can sometimes help when you are nervous and experiencing difficulty with direct eye contact.

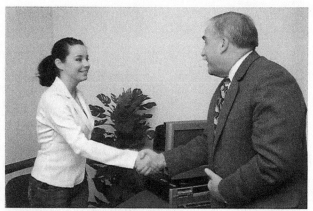

FIGURE 17-4A Shake hands firmly and smile when you greet an interviewer.

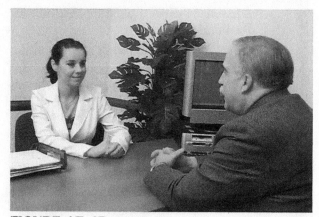

FIGURE 17-4B Sit straight and maintain eye contact during the interview.

♦ Listen closely to the interviewer. Do not interrupt in the middle of a sentence. Allow the interviewer to take the lead.

♦ Answer all questions thoroughly, but don't go into long, drawn-out explanations. Make sure your answers show how you are qualified for the job.

♦ Do *not* smoke, chew gum, or eat candy during the interview.

♦ Smile but avoid excessive laughter or giggling.

♦ Be yourself. Do not try to assume a different personality or different mannerisms; doing so will only increase your nervousness.

♦ Be enthusiastic. Display your positive attitude.

♦ Avoid awkward habits such as swinging your legs, jingling change in your pocket, waving your hands or arms, or patting at your hair.

◆ Never discuss personal problems, finances, or other situations in an effort to get the job. This usually has a negative effect on the interviewer.

◆ Do not criticize former employers or degrade them in any way.

◆ Answer all questions truthfully to the best of your ability.

◆ Think before you respond. Try to organize the information you present.

◆ Be proud of yourself, to a degree. You have skills and are trained. Make sure the interviewer is aware of this. However, be sure to show a willingness to learn and to gain additional knowledge.

◆ Do not immediately question the employer about salary, fringe benefits, insurance, and other similar items. This information is usually mentioned before the end of the interview. If the employer asks whether you have any questions, ask about the job description or responsibilities, type of uniform required, potential for career growth, continuing education or in-service programs, and job orientation. These types of questions indicate a sincere interest in the job rather than a "What's in it for me?" attitude.

◆ Do not expect a definite answer at the end of the interview. The interviewer will usually tell you that he or she will contact you.

◆ Thank the interviewer for the interview as you leave. If the interviewer extends a hand, shake hands firmly. Smile, be polite, and exit with confidence.

◆ Never try to extend the interview if the interviewer indicates that he or she is ready to end it.

After the interview, it is best to send a follow-up note, letter, or electronic message (e-mail) to thank the employer for the interview (figure 17-5). You may indicate that you are still interested in the position. You may also state that you are available for further questioning. When an employer is evaluating several applicants, a thank-you note is sometimes the deciding factor in who gets the job.

Because you may be asked many different questions during an interview, it is impossible to prepare all answers ahead of time. However, it is wise to think about some potential

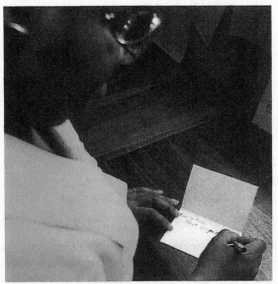

FIGURE 17-5 After a job interview, send a thank-you note, letter, or e-mail to the employer.

questions and your responses to them. The following is a suggested list of questions to review. Additional questions may be found in any book on job interviews.

◆ *Tell me a little about yourself.* (Note: Stick to job-related information.)

◆ *What are your strong points/weak points?* (Note: Be sure to turn a weakness into a positive point. For example, say, "One of my weaknesses is poor spelling, but I use a dictionary to check spelling and try to learn to spell ten new words each week.")

◆ *Why do you feel you are qualified for this position?*

◆ *What jobs have you held in the past? Why did you leave these jobs?* (Note: Avoid criticizing former employers.)

◆ *What school activities are you involved in?*

◆ *What kind of work interests you?*

◆ *Why do you want to work here?*

◆ *What skills do you have that would be of value?*

◆ *What is your attitude toward work?*

◆ *What do you want to know about this job opening?*

◆ *What were your favorite subjects in school and why?*

◆ *What does success mean to you?*

♦ *How do you manage your time?*

♦ *What is your image of the ideal job?*

♦ *How skilled are you with computers?*

♦ *What are the three most important things to you in a job?*

♦ *Do you prefer to work alone or with others? Why?*

♦ *How many days of school did you miss last year?*

♦ *What do you do in your spare time?*

♦ *Do you have any plans for further education?*

⚖ Any questions that may reflect discrimination or bias do *not* have to be answered during a job interview. Federal law prohibits discrimination with regard to age, cultural or ethnic background, marital status, parenthood, disability, religion, race, and sex. Employers are aware that it is illegal to ask questions of this nature, and the large majority will not ask such questions. If an employer does ask a question of this nature, however, you have the right to refuse to answer. An example of this type of question might be, "I see you married recently. Do you plan to start having children in the next year or two?" Be polite but firm in your refusal. A statement such as "I prefer not to answer that question" or "Can I ask you how this would affect the job we are discussing?" is usually sufficient.

⚖ At the end of the interview, you may be asked to provide proof of your eligibility to work. Under the Bureau of Immigration Reform Act of 1986, employers are now required by federal law to ask you to complete an Employment Eligibility Verification Form I-9. This form helps the employer verify that you are legally entitled to work in the United States. To complete this form, you must provide documents that indicate your identity. A birth certificate, passport, and/or immigration card can be used for this purpose. You must also have a photo identification, such as a driver's license, and a social security card. The employer must make copies of these documents and include them in your file. Having these forms readily available shows that you are prepared for a job.

STUDENT: *Go to the workbook and complete the assignment sheet for 17:4, Participating in a Job Interview. Then return and continue with the procedure.*

PROCEDURE 17:4

Participating in a Job Interview

Equipment and Supplies

Desk, two chairs, evaluation sheets, lists of questions

Procedure

1. Assemble equipment. Role-play a mock interview with four persons. Arrange for two people to evaluate the interview, one person to be the interviewer, and you to be the interviewee.

2. Position the two evaluators in such a way that they can observe both the interviewer and you, the person being interviewed. Make sure they will not interfere with the interview.

3. The interviewer should be seated at the desk and have a list of possible questions to ask during the interview.

4. Play the role of the person being interviewed. Prepare for this role by doing the following:

   a. Be sure you have all necessary information. Prepare your wallet card, résumé, job application form, and/or career passport or portfolio.

   b. Dress appropriately for the interview (as outlined in the preceding information section).

   c. Arrive at least 5–10 minutes early for the interview.

PROCEDURE 17:4

5. When you are called for the interview, introduce yourself. Be sure to refer to the interviewer by name.

6. Sit in the chair indicated. Be aware of your posture, making sure to sit straight. Keep your feet flat on the floor or cross your legs at the ankles only.

7. Listen closely to the employer. Answer all questions thoroughly and completely. Think before you speak. Organize your information.

8. Maintain eye contact. Avoid distracting mannerisms.

9. Use correct grammar. Avoid slang expressions. Speak in complete sentences. Practice good manners.

10. When you are asked whether you have any questions, ask questions pertaining to the job responsibilities. Avoid a series of questions on salary, fringe benefits, vacations, time off, and so forth.

11. At the end of the interview, thank the interviewer for his or her time. Shake hands as you leave.

12. Check your performance by looking at the evaluation sheets completed by the two observers. Study suggested changes.

13. Replace all equipment.

Practice

Go to the workbook and use the evaluation sheet for 17:4, Participating in a Job Interview, to practice this procedure. When you believe you have mastered this skill, sign the sheet and give it to your instructor for further action.

✔ **Final Checkpoint** Using the criteria listed on the evaluation sheet, your instructor will grade your performance.

17:5 INFORMATION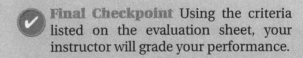

Determining Net Income

 Obtaining a job means, in part, that you will be earning your own money. This often means that you will be responsible for your own living expenses. To avoid debt and financial crisis, it is important that you learn about managing your money effectively, including understanding how to determine net income.

The term **income** usually means money that you earn or that is available to you. However, the amount you actually earn and the amount you receive to spend may vary. The following two terms explain the difference.

◆ **Gross income:** This is the total amount of money you earn for hours worked. It is the amount determined before any deductions have been taken out of your pay.

◆ **Net income:** This is commonly referred to as "take-home pay." It is the amount of money available to you after all payroll **deductions** have been taken out of your salary. Some common deductions are Social Security tax, federal and state taxes, and city taxes. Other deductions may include payroll deductions such as those for United Appeal, medical or life insurance, union dues, and other similar items.

To determine gross income, simply multiply your wage per hour times the number of hours worked. For example, if you earn $9.00 per hour and work a 40-hour week, $9 \times 40 = \$360.00$. In this example, then, $360.00 would be your gross income.

To determine net income, you must first determine the amounts of the various deductions that will be taken out of your gross pay. Deduc-

18   CHAPTER 1

tion percentages usually vary depending on your income level. You can usually determine approximate deduction percentages and, therefore, your approximate net income by referring to tax charts. Tax charts for federal taxes are available on the Internet at *www.irs.gov.* Tax charts for cities and states can usually be found on the treasurer's Internet site for the particular city or state. Never hesitate to ask your employer about deduction percentages. It is your responsibility to check your own paycheck for accuracy. Starting with the example of gross pay of $360.00, the following shows how net pay may be determined.

Gross Pay $360.00

◆ Deduction for federal tax in this income range is usually approximately 15 percent. Check tax tables for accuracy.

15%, or 0.15, × 360 = $54.00 $\frac{-54.00}{306.00}$

◆ Deduction for state tax is approximately 2 percent.

2%, or 0.02, × 360 = $7.20 $\frac{-7.20}{298.80}$

◆ Deduction for city tax is approximately 1 percent.

1%, or 0.01, × 360 = 3.60 $\frac{-3.60}{295.20}$

◆ Deduction for F.I.C.A., or Social Security tax, includes 6.2 percent of the first $102,000 in income and a Medicare deduction of 1.45 percent of the total in income, for a total deduction of 7.65 percent.

7.65%, or 0.0765, × 360 = 27.54 $\frac{-27.54}{267.66}$

◆ Net income after taxes, then, would be $267.66. Therefore, before you even receive your paycheck, $92.34 will be deducted from it. Additional deductions for insurance, union dues, contributions to charity, and other items may also be taken out of your gross pay.

In order to manage your money effectively, it is essential that you be able to calculate your net income. Because this is the amount of money you will have to spend, it will to some extent determine your lifestyle.

STUDENT: *Read and complete Procedure 17:5, Determining Net Income.*

PROCEDURE 17:5

Determining Net Income

Equipment and Supplies

Assignment sheet for 17:5, Determining Net Income; pen or pencil

Procedure

1. Assemble equipment. If a calculator is available, you may use it to complete this assignment.

2. Read the instructions on the assignment sheet in the workbook for 17:5, Determining Net Income. Use the assignment sheet with this procedure.

3. Determine your wage per hour by using your salary in a current job or an amount assigned by your instructor. Multiply this amount by the number of hours you work per week. This is your gross weekly pay.

4. If your instructor has federal tax tables, read the tax tables to determine the percentage, or amount of money, that will be withheld for federal tax. If tax tables are not available, look on the Internet at *www.irs.gov* or check with your employer to obtain this information.

    NOTE: The average withholding tax for an initial income bracket is usually approximately 15 percent. If you cannot find the exact amount or percentage, use this amount (0.15) for an approximate determination.

5. Multiply the percentage for federal tax times your gross weekly pay to deter-

PROCEDURE 17:5

mine the amount deducted for federal tax.

6. Determine the deduction for state tax by reading your state tax tables, checking the state treasurer's site on the Internet, or by consulting your employer.

   NOTE: An average state tax is 2 percent. If you cannot find the exact amount or percentage, use this amount (0.02) for an approximate determination.

7. Multiply the percentage for state tax by your gross weekly pay to determine the amount deducted for state tax.

8. Determine the deduction for any city or corporation tax by reading the city/corporation tax tables, checking the city/corporation treasurer's site on the Internet, or consulting your employer.

   NOTE: An average city/corporation tax is 1 percent. If you cannot find the exact amount or percentage, use this amount (0.01) for an approximate determination.

9. Multiply the percentage for city/corporation tax by your gross weekly pay to determine the amount deducted for city/corporation tax.

10. Check the current deduction for F.I.C.A., or Social Security and Medicare, by checking the Social Security Internet site or asking your employer for this information. Determine the deduction for F.I.C.A. by multiplying your gross weekly pay by this percentage.

    NOTE: In 2008, the F.I.C.A. rate was 6.2 percent of the first $102,000 in income and 1.45 percent of total income for Medicare. Use this total of 7.65 percent, or 0.0765, if you cannot obtain another percentage.

11. List the amounts for any other deductions. Examples include insurance, charitable donations, union dues, and similar items.

12. Add the amounts determined for federal tax, state tax, city/corporation tax, social security, and other deductions together.

13. Subtract the total amount for deductions from your gross weekly pay. The amount left is your net, or take-home, pay.

14. Recheck any figures, as needed.

15. Replace all equipment.

Practice

Go to the workbook and use the evaluation sheet for 17:5, Determining Net Income. Practice determining net income according to the criteria listed on the evaluation sheet. When you believe you have mastered this skill, sign the sheet and give it to your instructor for further action.

✓ **Final Checkpoint** Using the criteria listed on the evaluation sheet, your instructor will grade your performance.

17:6 INFORMATION

Calculating a Budget

 In order to use your net income wisely, it is best to prepare a budget. A **budget** is an itemized list of living expenses. It must be realistic to be effective.

A budget usually consists of two main types of expenses: fixed expenses and variable expenses. **Fixed expenses** include items such as rent or house payments, utilities, food, car payments, and insurance payments. **Variable expenses** include items such as entertainment, clothing purchases, and donations.

The easiest way to prepare a budget is to simply list all anticipated expenses for a one-month period. Then determine your net monthly pay. Allow a fair percentage of the net monthly pay for each of the budget items listed.

Savings should be incorporated into every budget. If saving money is regarded as an obligation, it is easier to set aside money for this purpose. When an emergency occurs, money is then available to cover the unexpected expenditure.

Some payments are due once or twice a year. An example is insurance payments. To be realistic, a monthly amount should be budgeted for this purpose. To determine a monthly amount, divide the total yearly cost for the insurance by 12. Then budget this amount each month. In this way, when insurance payments are due, the money is available for payment, and one month's budget will not have to bear the full amount of the insurance payment.

Money Management International (MMI), a nonprofit consumer counseling organization, recommends that the following percentage ranges of total net income be used while preparing a realistic budget:

- *Housing*: 20–35 percent
- *Food*: 15–30 percent
- *Utilities*: 4–7 percent
- *Transportation* (including car loan, insurance, gas, and maintenance): 6–20 percent
- *Insurance* (including health, life, and/or disability): 4–6 percent
- *Health* (including prescriptions, eye care, dental care): 2–8 percent
- *Clothing*: 3–10 percent
- *Personal care* (including soap, toothpaste, laundry detergents, cosmetics, etc.): 2–4 percent
- *Miscellaneous* (including travel, child care, entertainment, gifts, etc.): 1–4 percent
- *Savings*: 5–9 percent

It is important to remember that these percentages and line items are just suggested guidelines. Each individual must determine his or her own needs and allocate monies accordingly. However, MMI does state that personal debt should not exceed 10–20 percent of net income. Financial difficulties usually occur when debt exceeds this limit.

It is important that budgeted expenses do *not* exceed net monthly income. It may sometimes be necessary to limit expenses that are not fixed. Entertainment, clothing purchases, and similar items are examples of expenses that can be limited.

The final step is to live by your budget and avoid any spending over the allotted amounts. This is one way to prevent financial problems and excessive debt. If your fixed expenses or net income increases, you will have to revise your budget. Remember, creating a budget leads to careful management of hard-earned money.

STUDENT: *Read Procedure 17:6, Calculating a Budget. Then go to the workbook and complete the corresponding assignment sheet.*

PROCEDURE 17:6

Calculating a Budget

Equipment and Supplies

Assignment sheet for 17:6, Calculating a Budget; pen or pencil

Procedure

1. Assemble equipment. If a calculator is available, you may use it to complete this procedure.

2. Go to the workbook and read the instructions on the assignment sheet for 17:6, Calculating a Budget.

3. Determine your fixed expenses for a one-month period. This includes amounts you must pay for rent, utilities, loans, charge accounts, insurance, and similar items. List these expenses.

4. Determine your variable expenses for a one-month period. This includes amounts for clothing purchases, per-

PROCEDURE 17:6

sonal items, donations, entertainment, and similar items. List these expenses.

5. List any other items that must be included in your monthly budget. Be sure to list a reasonable amount for each item.

6. Determine a reasonable amount for savings. Many people prefer to set aside a certain percentage of their net monthly pay as savings.

7. Determine your net monthly pay. Double-check all figures for accuracy.

8. Add all of your monthly budget expenses together. The sum represents your total expenditures per month.

9. Compare your expense total to your net monthly income. If your expense total is higher than your net income, you will have to revise your budget and reduce any expenses that are not fixed. If your expense total is lower than your net income, you may increase the dollar amounts of your budget items. If the other figures in your budget are realistic, it may be wise to increase the dollar amount of savings.

10. When the expense total in your budget equals your monthly net income, you have a balanced budget. Live by this budget and avoid any expenditures not listed on the budget.

11. Replace all equipment.

Practice

Go to the workbook and use the evaluation sheet for 17:6, Calculating a Budget, to practice this procedure. When you believe you have mastered this skill, sign the sheet and give it to your instructor for further action. Give your instructor a completed budget along with the evaluation sheet.

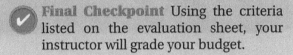 **Final Checkpoint** Using the criteria listed on the evaluation sheet, your instructor will grade your budget.

CHAPTER 17 SUMMARY

Even if an individual is proficient in many skills, it does not necessarily follow that the individual will obtain the "ideal" job. Just as it is important to learn the skills needed in your chosen health care career, it is important to learn the skills necessary to obtain a job.

Job-keeping skills important to an employer include using correct grammar in both oral and written communications, reporting to work on time and when scheduled, being prepared to work, following correct policies and procedures, having a positive attitude, working well with others, taking responsibility for your actions, and being willing to learn. Without good job-keeping skills, no amount of knowledge will help you keep a job.

One of the first steps in obtaining a job involves preparing a cover letter and a résumé. These are the "press releases" that tell a potential employer about your skills and abilities. A properly prepared résumé will help you obtain an interview.

It is important to prepare for an interview. Careful consideration should be given to dress and appearance. Answers should be prepared

TODAY'S RESEARCH: TOMORROW'S HEALTH CARE

A bravery gene?

Anxiety and fear have been felt by every human being. However, some individuals are so anxious or fearful they are not able to function within society. For example, individuals with agoraphobia have an abnormal fear of being helpless in a situation from which they cannot escape, so they stay in an environment in which they feel secure. Many agoraphobic people never leave their homes; they avoid all public or open places. Scientists are not really certain how fear works in the brain, so conditions such as these are difficult to treat.

Recently, scientists working with mice found that by removing a single gene, they could turn normally cautious animals into brave animals that were more willing to explore an unknown territory and were less intimidated by dangers. By analyzing brain tissue, scientists located a gene in a tiny prune-shaped region of the brain called the *amygdala*, an area of the brain that is extremely active when animals or humans are afraid or anxious. This gene produces a protein called *stathmin*, which is highly concentrated in the amygdala but very hard to detect in other areas of the brain. Scientists removed this stathmin gene and bred a line of mice that were all missing this gene. Tests showed that this breed of mice was twice as willing to explore unknown territories as unaltered mice. In addition, if the mice were trained to expect a small electrical shock after being presented with a stimulus such as a sound or sight, this group of mice did not seem as fearful when the sound or sight was given. Researchers are theorizing that stathmin helps form fearful memories in the amygdala of the brain, the area where unconscious fears seemed to be stored. If the production of stathmin could be halted or inhibited by medication, it is possible that fears would not be stored as unconscious memories. This would greatly decrease an individual's anxieties because unconscious fears are a major cause of anxiety. Think of all of the people whose lives are affected by anxiety and fear. If their anxieties and fears could be decreased or eliminated, they could lead normal healthy lives.

for common interview questions. The applicant should also try to learn as much as possible about the potential employer; this way, the applicant will be able to match his or her skills and abilities to the needs of the employer. Finally, practice completing job application forms. A neat, correct, and thorough application form will also help you get a job.

Certain other skills become essential when a person has a job. Everyone should be able to calculate gross and net income. In addition, everyone should be able to develop a budget based on needs and income. Having and following a budget makes it more likely that money earned will be spent wisely and minimizes the chance of debt. Learn the job-seeking and job-keeping skills well. They will benefit you throughout your life as you seek new positions of employment and advance in your chosen health career.

INTERNET SEARCHES

Use the suggested search engines in Chapter 12:4 of this textbook to search the Internet for additional information on the following topics:

1. *Components of a job search*: find information on letters of application or cover letters, résumés, job interviews, and job application forms

3. *Requirements of employers*: locate information on skills and qualities that employers desire

4. *Job search*: look for sites that provide information on employment opportunities. For specific health care careers, look for opportunities under organizations for the specific career. Also check general sites such as *monster.com, job-listing.com, jobsleuth.com, hotjobs.yahoo. com, careerbuilder.com,* and *joblocator.com.*

4. *Salary and wages*: check sites such as the Internal Revenue Service (IRS), state and local tax departments, and Social Security Administration for information on taxes and tax rates; also locate sites on money management, budgeting, and fiscal or financial management for information on how to manage money

REVIEW QUESTIONS

1. Choose four (4) job-keeping skills that you believe you have mastered. Write a paragraph describing why you believe you have mastered these skills.

2. What is the main purpose of a letter of application or cover letter? When is it used?

3. List the main sections of a résumé and briefly describe the information that should be included in each section.

4. State six (6) basic principles that must be followed while completing a job application form.

5. Create answers for the following interview questions.
   a. Why do you believe you are qualified for this job?
   b. Why do you want to leave your current job?
   c. Tell me about two or three of your major accomplishments and why you feel they are important.

6. You have obtained a job and will receive a salary of $8.20 per hour. Calculate the following:
   a. Gross pay for a 40-hour week
   b. Federal tax deduction of 15%
   c. State tax deduction of 3%
   d. City tax deduction of 0.5%
   e. FICA or social security deduction of 7.65%
   f. Net pay after above deductibles

CHAPTER 2

Infection Control

Introduction

After completing this unit of study, you should be able to:

◆ Identify five classes of microorganisms by describing the characteristics of each class
◆ List the six components of the chain of infection
◆ Differentiate between antisepsis, disinfection, and sterilization
◆ Wash hands according to recommended aseptic technique
◆ Observe standard precautions while working in the laboratory or clinical area
◆ Wash, wrap, and autoclave instruments, linen, and equipment
◆ Operate an autoclave with accuracy and safety
◆ Follow basic principles on using chemicals for disinfection
◆ Clean instruments with an ultrasonic unit
◆ Open sterile packages without contaminating the contents
◆ Don sterile gloves without contaminating the gloves
◆ Prepare a sterile dressing tray without contaminating the supplies
◆ Change a sterile dressing without contaminating the materials
◆ Don and remove a transmission-based isolation mask, gloves, and gown
◆ Relate specific basic tasks to the care of a patient in a transmission-based isolation unit
◆ Define, pronounce, and spell all the key terms

 Observe Standard Precautions

 Safety—Proceed with Caution

 Math Skill

 Science Skill

C Communications Skill

 Instructors Check—Call Instructor at This Point

 OBRA Requirement— Based on Federal Law

 Legal Responsibility

 Career Information

 Technology

KEY TERMS

acquired immune deficiency
  syndrome (AIDS)
aerobic
airborne precautions
anaerobic
antisepsis
  (ant"-ih-sep'-sis)
asepsis
  (a-sep'-sis)
autoclave
bacteria
causative agent
cavitation
  (kav"-ih-tay'-shun)
chain of infection
chemical disinfection
clean
communicable disease
contact precautions

contaminated
disinfection
droplet precautions
endogenous
exogenous
fomites
fungi
  (fun'-guy)
hepatitis B
hepatitis C
microorganism
  (my-crow-or'-gan-izm)
mode of transmission
nonpathogens
nosocomial
opportunistic
pathogens
  (path'-oh-jenz")

personal protective equipment
  (PPE)
portal of entry
portal of exit
protective (reverse) isolation
protozoa
  (pro-toe-zo'-ah)
reservoir
rickettsiae
  (rik-et'-z-ah)
standard precautions
sterile
sterile field
sterilization
susceptible host
transmission-based isolation
  precautions
ultrasonic
viruses

13:1 INFORMATION Understanding the Principles of Infection Control

OBRA Understanding the basic principles of infection control is essential for any health care worker in any field of health care. The principles described in this unit provide a basic knowledge of how disease is transmitted and the main ways to prevent disease transmission.

A **microorganism,** or microbe, is a small, living organism that is not visible to the naked eye. It must be viewed under a microscope. Microorganisms are found everywhere in the environment, including on and in the human body. Many microorganisms are part of the normal flora (plant life adapted for living in a specific environment) of the body and are beneficial in

maintaining certain body processes. These are called **nonpathogens.** Other microorganisms cause infection and disease and are called **pathogens,** or germs. At times, a microorganism that is beneficial in one body system can become pathogenic when it is present in another body system. For example, a bacterium called *Escherichia coli* (*E. coli*) is part of the natural flora of the large intestine. If *E. coli* enters the urinary system, however, it causes an infection.

There are many different classes of microorganisms. In each class, some of the microorganisms are pathogenic to humans. The main classes include:

◆ **Bacteria**—These are simple, one-celled organisms that multiply rapidly. They are classified by shape and arrangement. *Cocci* are round or spherical in shape (see figure 13-1). If cocci occur in pairs, they are diplococci. Diplococci bacteria cause diseases such as gonorrhea, meningitis, and pneumonia. If cocci occur in chains, they are streptococci. A common streptococcus causes a severe sore throat (strep throat) and rheumatic fever. If

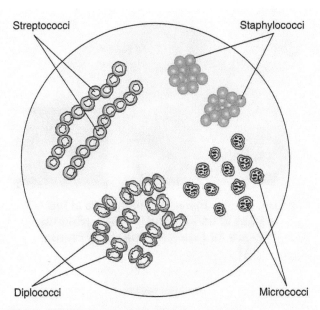

FIGURE 13-1 Kinds of cocci bacteria.

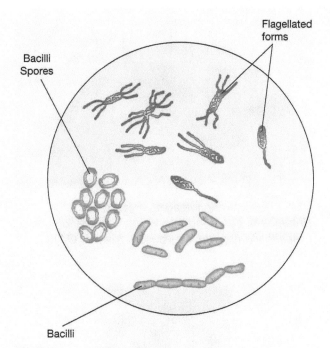

FIGURE 13-2 Bacilli bacteria.

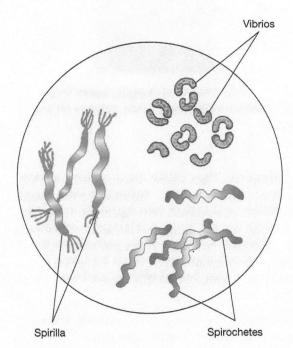

FIGURE 13-3 Spirilla bacteria.

cocci occur in clusters or groups, they are staphylococci. These are the most common pyogenic (pus-producing) microorganisms. Staphylococci cause infections such as boils, wound infections, and toxic shock. Rod-shaped bacteria are called *bacilli* (see figure 13-2). They can occur singly, in pairs, or in chains. Many bacilli contain flagella, which are threadlike projections that are similar to tails and allow the organisms to move. Bacilli also have the ability to form spores, or thick-walled capsules, when conditions for growth are poor. In the spore form, bacilli are extremely difficult to kill. Diseases caused by different types of bacilli include tuberculosis; tetanus; pertussis, or whooping cough; botulism; diphtheria; and typhoid. Bacteria that are spiral or corkscrew in shape are called *spirilla* (see figure 13-3). These include the comma-shaped vibrio and the corkscrew-shaped spirochete. Diseases caused by spirilla include syphilis and cholera. Antibiotics are used to kill bacteria. However, some strains of bacteria have become antibiotic-resistant, which means that the antibiotic is no longer effective against the bacteria.

◆ **Protozoa**—These are one-celled animal-like organisms often found in decayed materials and contaminated water (see figure 13-4). Many contain flagella which allow them to move freely. Some protozoa are pathogenic and cause diseases such as malaria, amebic

dysentery, trichomonas, and African sleeping sickness.

◆ **Fungi**—These are simple, plant-like organisms that live on dead organic matter. Yeasts and molds are two common forms that can be

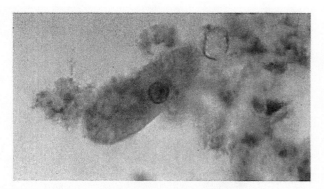

FIGURE 13-4 An intestinal protozoan, *Entamoeba coli. (Courtesy of the Centers for Disease Control and Prevention, Atlanta, GA)*

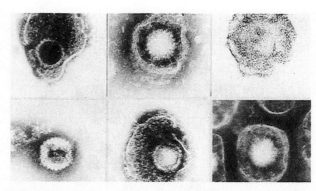

FIGURE 13-6A Electron micrographs of the various types of herpes simplex virus. *(Courtesy of the Centers for Disease Control and Prevention, Atlanta, GA)*

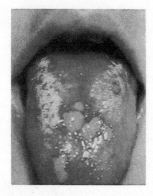

FIGURE 13-5 The yeast (fungus) called thrush causes these characteristic white patches on the tongue.

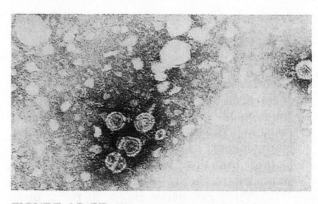

FIGURE 13-6B Electron micrograph of the hepatitis B virus. *(Courtesy of the Centers for Disease Control and Prevention, Atlanta, GA)*

pathogenic. They cause diseases such as ringworm, athlete's foot, histoplasmosis, yeast vaginitis, and thrush (see figure 13-5). Antibiotics do not kill fungi. Antifungal medications are available for many of the pathogenic fungi, but they are expensive, must be taken internally for a long period of time, and may cause liver damage.

◆ **Rickettsiae**—These are parasitic microorganisms, which means they cannot live outside the cells of another living organism. They are commonly found in fleas, lice, ticks, and mites and are transmitted to humans by the bites of these insects. Rickettsiae cause diseases such as typhus fever and Rocky Mountain spotted fever. Antibiotics are effective against many different rickettsiae.

◆ **OBRA** **Viruses**—These are the smallest microorganisms, visible only using an electron microscope (see figure 13-6A and B). They cannot reproduce unless they are inside another living cell. They are spread from human to human by blood and other body secretions. It is important to note that viruses are more difficult to kill because they are resistant to many disinfectants and are not affected by antibiotics. Viruses cause many diseases including the common cold, measles, mumps, chicken pox, herpes, warts, influenza, and polio. Three diseases of major concern to the health care worker are hepatitis B, hepatitis C, and acquired immune deficiency syndrome (AIDS). **Hepatitis B,** or serum hepatitis, is caused by the HBV virus and is transmitted by blood, serum, and other body secretions. It affects the liver and can lead to the destruction and scarring of liver cells. A vaccine has been developed to protect individuals from this disease. The vaccine is expensive and involves a series of three injections. Under federal law, employers must provide the vaccination at no cost to any health care worker with occupational exposure to blood or other body secretions that may carry the HBV virus. An individual does have the right to refuse the vaccination, but a written record must be kept proving that the vaccine was offered. **Hepatitis C** is caused by the hepatitis C virus, or HCV, and is transmitted by blood and blood-containing body fluids. Many individuals who contact the disease are asymptomatic (display no symptoms); others have mild symptoms that are often diagnosed as influenza or flu. In either case, HCV can cause serious liver damage. At present there is no preventive immunization, but a vaccine is being developed. Both HBV and HCV are extremely difficult to destroy. These viruses can even remain active for several days in dried blood. Health care workers must take every precaution to protect themselves from hepatitis viruses. **Acquired immune deficiency syndrome** is caused by the human immunodeficiency virus (HIV) and suppresses the immune system. An individual with AIDS cannot fight off many cancers and infections that would not affect a healthy person. Presently there is no cure and no vaccine available, so it is important for the health care worker to take precautions to prevent the spread of this disease.

In order to grow and reproduce, microorganisms need certain things. Most microorganisms prefer a warm environment, and body temperature is ideal. Darkness is also preferred by most microorganisms, and many are killed quickly by sunlight. In addition, a source of food and moisture is needed. Some microorganisms, called **aerobic** organisms, require oxygen to live. Others, called **anaerobic** organisms, live and reproduce in the absence of oxygen. The human body is the ideal supplier of all the requirements of microorganisms.

Pathogenic microorganisms cause infection and disease in different ways. Some pathogens produce poisons, called *toxins,* which harm the body. An example is the bacillus that causes tetanus, which produces toxins that damage the central nervous system. Some pathogens cause an allergic reaction in the body, resulting in a runny nose, watery eyes, and sneezing. Other pathogens attack and destroy the living cells they invade. An example is the protozoan that causes malaria. It invades red blood cells and causes them to rupture.

Infections and diseases are also classified as endogenous, exogenous, nosocomial, or opportunistic. **Endogenous** means the infection or disease originates within the body. These include metabolic disorders, congenital abnormalities, tumors, and infections caused by microorganisms within the body. **Exogenous** means the infection or disease originates outside the body. Examples include pathogenic organisms that invade the body, radiation, chemical agents, trauma, electric shock, and temperature extremes. A **nosocomial** infection is one acquired by an individual in a health care facility such as a hospital or long-term care facility. Nosocomial infections are usually present in the facility and transmitted by health care workers to the patient. Many of the pathogens transmitted in this manner are antibiotic-resistant and can cause serious and even life-threatening infections in patients. Common examples are staphylococcus, pseudomonas, and enterococci. Infection-control programs are used in health care facilities to prevent and deal with nosocomial infections. **Opportunistic** infections are those that occur when the body's defenses are weak. These diseases do not usually occur in individuals with intact immune systems. Examples include the development of Kaposi's sarcoma (a rare type of cancer) or *Pneumocystis carinii* pneumonia in individuals with AIDS.

In order for disease to occur and spread from one individual to another, certain conditions must be met. First, there must be a **causative agent,** or pathogen, such as a bacterium or virus. Second, the causative agent must find a **reservoir** where it can live. Some common reservoirs include the human body, animals, the environment, and **fomites,** or objects contaminated with infectious material that contains the pathogens. Common fomites include doorknobs, bedpans, urinals, linens, instruments, and specimen containers. The pathogen must then have a **portal of exit,** or a way to escape from the reservoir in which it has been growing. In the human body, pathogens can leave the body through urine, feces, saliva, blood, tears, mucous discharge, sexual secretions, and draining wounds. When the pathogen leaves the reservoir, it must have a **mode of transmission,** or way in which it can be transmitted to another reservoir or host where it can live. The pathogen can be transmitted in different ways. One way is by direct person-to-person contact (physical or sexual contact), or direct contact with a body secretion containing the pathogen. Contaminated hands are one of the most common sources of direct transmission. Another way is by indirect contact, when the pathogen is transmitted from contaminated substances such as food, air, soil, insects, feces, clothing, instruments, and equipment. Examples include touching contaminated equipment and spreading the pathogen on the hands, breathing in droplets carrying airborne infections, and being bitten by an insect carrying a pathogen. A **portal of entry,** or a way to enter a new reservoir or host, is also essential. Some ways pathogens can enter the body are through breaks in the skin, breaks in the mucous membrane, the respiratory tract, the digestive tract, the genitourinary tract, and the circulatory system. If the defense mechanisms of the body are intact and the immune system is functioning, a human can frequently fight off the causative agent and not contract the disease. Body defenses include:

- *mucous membrane:* lines the respiratory, digestive, and reproductive tracts and traps pathogens;
- *cilia:* tiny, hairlike structures that line the respiratory tract and propel pathogens out of the body;
- *coughing and sneezing;*
- *hydrochloric acid:* destroys pathogens in the stomach;
- *tears in the eye:* contain bacteriocidal (killing bacteria) chemicals;
- *fever;*
- *inflammation:* leukocytes, or white blood cells, destroy pathogens;
- *immune response:* body produces antibodies, protective proteins that combat pathogens, and protective chemicals secreted by cells, such as interferon and complement.

However, if large numbers of a pathogen invade the body, or if the body defenses are weak, the individual can contract the infection or disease. This individual is called a **susceptible host,** or a person likely to get an infection or disease. These factors—a causative agent, a reservoir, a portal of exit, a mode of transmission, a portal of entry, and a susceptible host—form what is commonly called the **chain of infection** (see figure 13-7). If any part of the chain is eliminated, the spread of disease or infection will be stopped. A health care worker who is aware of this can follow practices to interrupt or break this chain and prevent the transmission of disease. It is important to remember that pathogens are everywhere and that preventing their transmission is a continuous process.

A major way to break the chain of infection is to use aseptic techniques while providing health care. **Asepsis** is defined as the absence of disease-producing microorganisms, or pathogens. Any object or area that may contain pathogens is considered to be contaminated. Aseptic techniques are directed toward maintaining cleanliness and eliminating or preventing contamination. Common aseptic techniques include handwashing, good personal hygiene, use of disposable gloves when contacting body secretions or contaminated objects, proper cleaning of instruments and equipment, and thorough cleaning of the environment.

Various levels of aseptic control are possible. These include:

- **Antisepsis**—Antiseptics prevent or inhibit growth of pathogenic organisms but are not effective against spores and viruses. They can usually be used on the skin. Common examples include alcohol and betadine.

- **Disinfection**—This is a process that destroys or kills pathogenic organisms. It is not always effective against spores and viruses. Chemical disinfectants are used in this process. Disinfectants can irritate or damage the skin and are used mainly on objects, not people. Some common disinfectants are bleach solutions and zephirin.

- **Sterilization**—This is a process that destroys all microorganisms, both pathogenic and non-pathogenic, including spores and viruses. Steam under pressure, gas, radiation, and chemicals can be used to sterilize objects. An autoclave is the most common piece of equipment used for sterilization.

In the sections that follow, correct methods of aseptic techniques are described. It is important for the health care worker to know and use these methods in every aspect of providing health care in order to prevent the spread and transmission of disease.

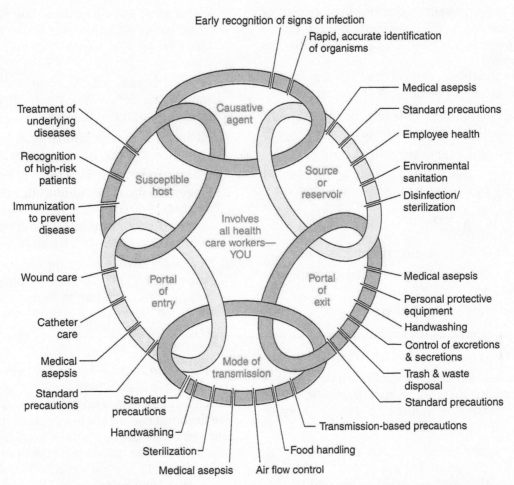

FIGURE 13-7 Note the components in the chain of infection and the ways in which the chain can be broken.

STUDENT: *Go to the workbook and complete the assignment sheet for 13:1, Understanding the Principles of Infection Control.*

13:2 INFORMATION Washing Hands

⊛ OBRA Handwashing is a basic task required in any health occupation. The method described in this unit has been developed to ensure that a thorough cleansing occurs. An aseptic technique is a method followed to prevent the spread of germs or pathogens. *Handwashing is the most important method used to practice aseptic technique.* Handwashing is also the most effective way to prevent the spread of infection.

The hands are a perfect medium for the spread of pathogens. Thoroughly washing the hands helps prevent and control the spread of pathogens from one person to another. It also helps protect the health worker from disease and illness.

Handwashing should be performed frequently. It should be done:

- When you arrive at the facility and immediately before leaving the facility
- Before and after every patient contact
- Any time the hands become contaminated during a procedure
- Before applying and immediately after removing gloves
- Before and after handling any specimen
- After contact with any soiled or contaminated item
- After picking up any item off the floor
- After personal use of the bathroom
- After you cough, sneeze, or use a tissue
- Before and after any contact with your mouth or mucous membrane, such as eating, drinking, smoking, applying lip balm, or inserting or removing contact lenses

The recommended method for handwashing is based on the following principles; they should be observed whenever hands are washed:

- Soap is used as a cleansing agent because it aids in the removal of germs through its sudsy action and alkali content. Pathogens are trapped in the soapsuds and rinsed away. Use liquid soap from a dispenser whenever possible because bar soap can contain microorganisms.

- Warm water should be used. This is less damaging to the skin than hot water. It also creates a better lather with soap than does cold water.
- Friction must be used in addition to soap and water. This action helps rub off pathogens from the surface of the skin.
- All surfaces on the hands must be cleaned. This includes the palms, the backs/tops of the hands, and the areas between the fingers.
- Fingertips must be pointed downward. The downward direction prevents water from getting on the forearms and then running down to contaminate the clean hands.
- Dry paper towels must be used to turn the faucet on and off. This action prevents contamination of the hands from pathogens on the faucet. A dry towel must be used because pathogens can travel more readily through a wet towel.

Nails also harbor dirt and must be cleaned during the handwashing process. An orange/cuticle stick can be used. Care must be taken to use the blunt end of the stick because the pointed end can injure the nailbeds. A brush can also be used to clean the nails. If a brush or orange stick is not available, the nails can be rubbed against the palm of the opposite hand. Keep the nails short to prevent scratching the skin.

STUDENT: *Go to the workbook and complete the assignment sheet for 13:2, Washing Hands. Then return and continue with the procedure.*

PROCEDURE 13:2

Washing Hands

Equipment and Supplies

Paper towels, running water, waste container, hand brush or orange/cuticle stick, soap

Procedure

1. Assemble all equipment. Stand back slightly from the sink so you do not contaminate

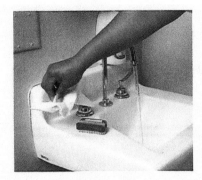

FIGURE 13-8A Use a dry towel to turn the faucet on.

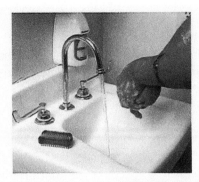

FIGURE 13-8B Point the fingertips downward and use the palm of one hand to clean the back of the other hand.

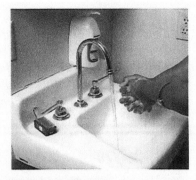

FIGURE 13-8C Interlace the fingers to clean between the fingers.

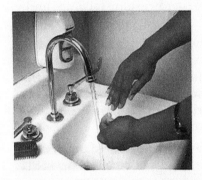

FIGURE 13-8D The blunt end of an orange stick can be used to clean the nails.

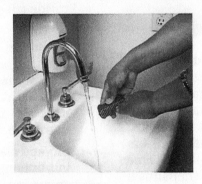

FIGURE 13-8E A hand brush can also be used to clean the nails.

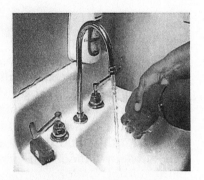

FIGURE 13-8F With the fingertips pointing downward, rinse the hands thoroughly.

your uniform or clothing. Avoid touching the inside of the sink with your hands since it is considered contaminated.

2. Turn the faucet on by holding a paper towel between your hand and the faucet (see figure 13-8A). Regulate the temperature of the water and let water flow over your hands. Discard the towel in the waste container.
   NOTE: Water should be warm.
   ⚠ **CAUTION:** Hot water will burn your hands.

3. With your fingertips pointing downward, wet your hands.
   NOTE: Washing in a downward direction prevents water from getting on the forearms and then running back down to contaminate hands.

4. Use soap to get a lather on your hands.

5. Put the palms of your hands together and rub them using friction and a circular motion for approximately 10 to 15 seconds.

6. Put the palm of one hand on the back of the other hand. Rub together several times.

Repeat this after reversing position of hands (see figure 13-8B).

7. Interlace the fingers on both hands and rub them back and forth (see figure 13-8C).

8. Clean the nails with an orange/cuticle stick and/or hand brush (see figures 13-8D and E).
   ⚠ **CAUTION:** Use the blunt end of orange/cuticle stick to avoid injury.
   NOTE: Steps 3 through 8 ensure that all parts of both hands are clean.

9. Rinse your hands, keeping fingertips pointed downward (see figure 13-8F).

10. Use a clean paper towel to dry hands thoroughly, from tips of fingers to wrist. Discard the towel in the waste container.

11. Use another dry paper towel to turn off the faucet.
    ⚠ **CAUTION:** Wet towels allow passage of pathogens.

12. Discard all used towels in the waste container. Leave the area neat and clean.

Practice *Go to the workbook and use the evaluation sheet for 13:2, Washing Hands, to practice this procedure. When you feel you have mastered this skill, sign the sheet and give it to your instructor for further action.*

✔ **Final Checkpoint** Using the criteria listed on the evaluation sheet, your instructor will grade your performance.

13:3 INFORMATION Observing Standard Precautions

 OBRA In order to prevent the spread of pathogens and disease, the chain of infection must be broken. The standard precautions discussed in this unit are an important way health care workers can break this chain.

One of the main ways that pathogens are spread is by blood and body fluids. Three pathogens of major concern are the hepatitis B virus (HBV), the hepatitis C virus (HCV), and the human immunodeficiency virus (HIV), which causes AIDS. Consequently, extreme care must be taken at all times when an area, object, or person is contaminated with blood or body fluids. In 1991, the Occupational Safety and Health Administration (OSHA) established *Bloodborne Pathogen Standards* that must be followed by all health care facilities. The employer faces civil penalties if the regulations are not implemented by the employer and followed by the employees. These regulations require all health care facility employers to:

- Develop a written exposure control plan, and update it annually, to minimize or eliminate employee exposure to bloodborne pathogens.

- Identify all employees who have occupational exposure to blood or potentially infectious materials such as semen, vaginal secretions, and other body fluids.

- Provide hepatitis B vaccine free of charge to all employees who have occupational exposure, and obtain a written release form signed by any employee who does not want the vaccine.

- Provide **personal protective equipment (PPE)** such as gloves, gowns, lab coats, masks, and face shields in appropriate sizes and in accessible locations.

- Provide adequate handwashing facilities and supplies.

- Ensure that the worksite is maintained in a clean and sanitary condition, follow measures for immediate decontamination of any surface that comes in contact with blood or infectious materials, and dispose of infectious waste correctly.

- Enforce rules of no eating, drinking, smoking, applying cosmetics or lip balm, handling contact lenses, and mouth pipetting or suctioning in any area that can be potentially contaminated by blood or other body fluids.

- Provide appropriate containers that are color coded (fluorescent orange or orange-red) and labeled for contaminated sharps (needles, scalpels) and other infectious or biohazard wastes.

- Post signs at the entrance to work areas where there is occupational exposure to biohazardous materials.

- Provide a confidential medical evaluation and follow-up for any employee who has an exposure incident. Examples might include an accidental needle stick or the splashing of blood or body fluids on the skin, eyes, or mucous membranes.

- Provide training about the regulations and all potential biohazards to all employees at no cost during working hours, and provide additional education as needed when procedures or working conditions are changed or modified.

In 2001, OSHA revised its Bloodborne Pathogen Standards in response to Congress passing the *Needlestick Safety and Prevention*

Act in November, 2000. This act was passed after the Centers for Disease Control and Prevention (CDC) estimated that 600,000 to 800,000 needle sticks occur each year, exposing health care workers to bloodborne pathogens. Employers are required to:

◆ *Identify and use effective and safer medical devices:* OSHA defines safer devices as sharps with engineered injury protections and includes, but is not limited to, devices such as syringes with a sliding sheath that shields the needle after use, needles that retract into a syringe after use, shielded or retracting catheters that can be used to administer intravenous medications or fluids, and intravenous systems that administer medication or fluids through a catheter port or connector site using a needle housed in a protective covering (see figure 13-9). OSHA also encourages the use of needleless systems which include, but are not limited to, intravenous medication delivery systems that administer medication or fluids through a catheter port or connector site using a blunt cannula or other non-needle connection, and jet injection systems that deliver subcutaneous or intramuscular injections through the skin without using a needle.

◆ *Incorporate changes in annual update of Exposure Control Plan:* Employers must include changes in technology that eliminate or reduce exposure to bloodborne pathogens in the annual update and document the implementation of any safer medical devices.

◆ *Solicit input from nonmanagerial employees who are responsible for direct patient care:* Employees who provide patient care, and are exposed to injuries from contaminated sharps, must be included in a multidisciplinary team that identifies, evaluates, and selects safer medical devices, and determines safer work practice controls.

◆ *Maintain a sharps injury log:* Employers with more than 11 employees must maintain a sharps injury log to help identify high risk areas and evaluate ways of decreasing injuries. Each injury recorded must protect the confidentiality of the injured employee, but must state the type and brand of device involved in the incident, the work area or department where the exposure injury

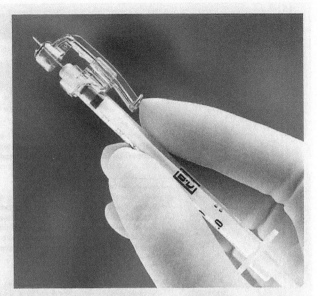

FIGURE 13-9 The Safety-Glide syringe is one example of a safer device to prevent needlesticks. *(Photo reprinted courtesy of BD [Becton Dickinson and Company])*

occurred, and a description of how the incident occurred.

Employers are also required to make sure that every employee uses standard precautions at all times to prevent contact with blood or other potentially infectious materials. **Standard precautions** (see figure 13-10) are rules developed by the Centers for Disease Control and Prevention (CDC). According to standard precautions, every body fluid must be considered a potentially infectious material, and all patients must be considered potential sources of infection, regardless of their disease or diagnosis. Standard precautions must be used in any situation where health care providers may contact:

◆ Blood or any fluid that may contain blood

◆ Body fluids, secretions, and excretions, such as mucus, sputum, saliva, cerebrospinal fluid, urine, feces, vomitus, amniotic fluid (surrounding a fetus), synovial (joint) fluid, pleural (lung) fluid, pericardial (heart) fluid, peritoneal (abdominal cavity) fluid, semen, and vaginal secretions

◆ Mucous membranes

◆ Nonintact skin

◆ Tissue or cell specimens

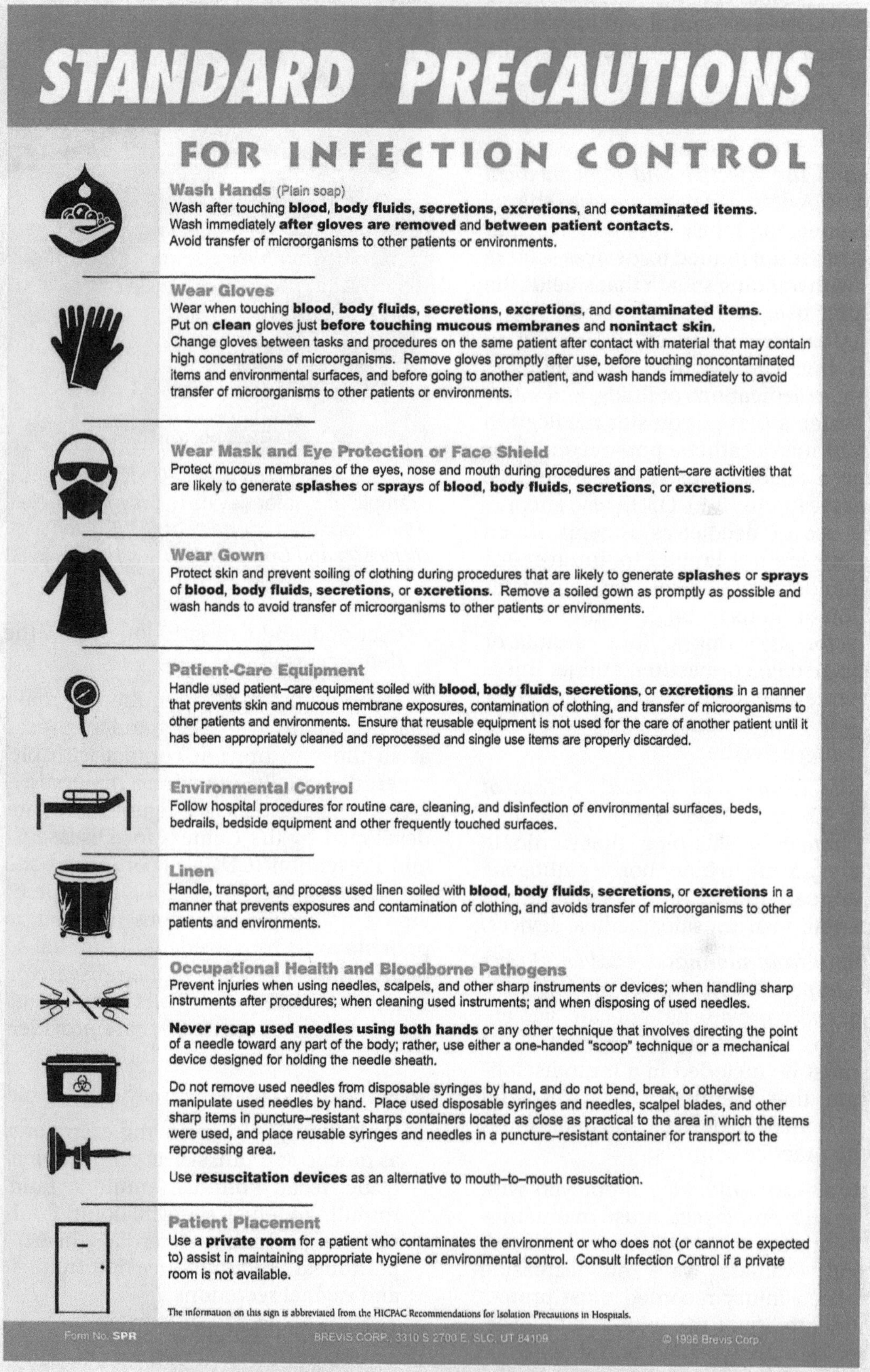

STANDARD PRECAUTIONS

FOR INFECTION CONTROL

Wash Hands (Plain soap)
Wash after touching **blood**, **body fluids**, **secretions**, **excretions**, and **contaminated items**.
Wash immediately **after gloves are removed** and **between patient contacts**.
Avoid transfer of microorganisms to other patients or environments.

Wear Gloves
Wear when touching **blood**, **body fluids**, **secretions**, **excretions**, and **contaminated items**.
Put on **clean** gloves just **before touching mucous membranes** and **nonintact skin**.
Change gloves between tasks and procedures on the same patient after contact with material that may contain
high concentrations of microorganisms. Remove gloves promptly after use, before touching noncontaminated
items and environmental surfaces, and before going to another patient, and wash hands immediately to avoid
transfer of microorganisms to other patients or environments.

Wear Mask and Eye Protection or Face Shield
Protect mucous membranes of the eyes, nose and mouth during procedures and patient–care activities that
are likely to generate **splashes** or **sprays** of **blood**, **body fluids**, **secretions**, or **excretions**.

Wear Gown
Protect skin and prevent soiling of clothing during procedures that are likely to generate **splashes** or **sprays**
of **blood**, **body fluids**, **secretions**, or **excretions**. Remove a soiled gown as promptly as possible and
wash hands to avoid transfer of microorganisms to other patients or environments.

Patient-Care Equipment
Handle used patient–care equipment soiled with **blood**, **body fluids**, **secretions**, or **excretions** in a manner
that prevents skin and mucous membrane exposures, contamination of clothing, and transfer of microorganisms to
other patients and environments. Ensure that reusable equipment is not used for the care of another patient until it
has been appropriately cleaned and reprocessed and single use items are properly discarded.

Environmental Control
Follow hospital procedures for routine care, cleaning, and disinfection of environmental surfaces, beds,
bedrails, bedside equipment and other frequently touched surfaces.

Linen
Handle, transport, and process used linen soiled with **blood**, **body fluids**, **secretions**, or **excretions** in a
manner that prevents exposures and contamination of clothing, and avoids transfer of microorganisms to other
patients and environments.

Occupational Health and Bloodborne Pathogens
Prevent injuries when using needles, scalpels, and other sharp instruments or devices; when handling sharp
instruments after procedures; when cleaning used instruments; and when disposing of used needles.

Never recap used needles using both hands or any other technique that involves directing the point
of a needle toward any part of the body; rather, use either a one-handed "scoop" technique or a mechanical
device designed for holding the needle sheath.

Do not remove used needles from disposable syringes by hand, and do not bend, break, or otherwise
manipulate used needles by hand. Place used disposable syringes and needles, scalpel blades, and other
sharp items in puncture–resistant sharps containers located as close as practical to the area in which the items
were used, and place reusable syringes and needles in a puncture–resistant container for transport to the
reprocessing area.

Use **resuscitation devices** as an alternative to mouth–to–mouth resuscitation.

Patient Placement
Use a **private room** for a patient who contaminates the environment or who does not (or cannot be expected
to) assist in maintaining appropriate hygiene or environmental control. Consult Infection Control if a private
room is not available.

The information on this sign is abbreviated from the HICPAC Recommendations for Isolation Precautions in Hospitals.

Form No. **SPR**   BREVIS CORP. 3310 S 2700 E, SLC, UT 84109   © 1996 Brevis Corp.

FIGURE 13-10 Standard precautions must be observed while working with all patients.
(Courtesy of Brevis Corporation)

A major precaution is to wash your hands before and after contact with any patient. If your hands or other skin surfaces are contaminated with blood, body fluids, secretions, or excretions, they must be washed immediately and thoroughly with soap and water. Hands must always be washed immediately after removal of gloves.

Gloves (see figure 13-11) must be worn whenever contact with blood, body fluids, secretions, excretions, mucous membranes, tissue specimens, or nonintact skin is possible; when handling or cleaning any contaminated items or surfaces; when performing any invasive (entering the body) procedure; and when performing venipuncture or blood tests. Rings must be removed before putting on gloves to avoid puncturing the gloves. Gloves must be changed after contact with each patient, and hands must be washed immediately after removal of gloves. Care must be taken while removing gloves to avoid contamination of the skin. Gloves must *not* be washed or disinfected for reuse because washing may allow penetration of liquids through undetected holes, and disinfecting agents may cause deterioration of gloves.

Gowns must be worn during any procedure that is likely to cause splashing or spraying of blood, body fluids, secretions, or excretions. This helps prevent contamination of clothing or uniforms. Contaminated gowns must be handled according to agency policy and local and state laws. Wash hands immediately after removing a gown.

Masks and protective eyewear or face shields (see figure 13-12) must be worn during procedures that may produce splashes or sprays of blood, body fluids, secretions, or excretions. Examples include irrigation of wounds, suctioning, dental procedures, delivery of a baby, and surgical procedures. This prevents exposure of the mucous membranes of the mouth, nose,

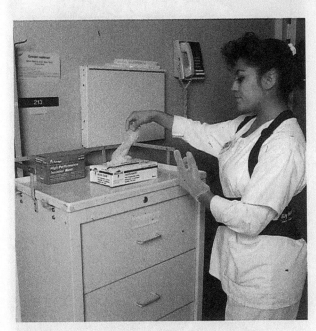

FIGURE 13-11 Gloves must be worn whenever contact with blood, body fluids, secretions, excretions, mucous membranes, or nonintact skin is possible.

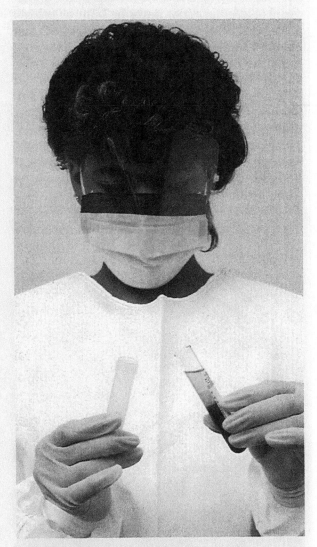

FIGURE 13-12 Gloves, a gown, a mask, and protective eyewear must be worn during any procedure that may produce droplets or cause splashing of blood, body fluids, secretions, or excretions.

and eyes to any pathogens. Masks must be used once and then discarded. In addition, masks should be changed every 30 minutes or anytime they become moist or wet. They should be removed by grasping the ties or elastic strap. Hands must be washed immediately after the mask is removed. Protective eyewear or face shields should provide protection for the front, top, bottom, and sides of the eyes. If eyewear is not disposable, it must be cleaned and disinfected before it is reused.

To avoid accidental cuts or punctures, extreme care must be taken while handling sharp objects. Whenever possible, safe needles or needleless devices must be used. Disposable needles must never be bent or broken after use. They must be left uncapped and attached to the syringe and placed in a leakproof puncture-resistant sharps container (see figure 13-13). The sharps container must be labeled with a red biohazard symbol (see figure 13-14). Surgical blades, razors, and other sharp objects must also be discarded in the sharps container. The containers must *not* be emptied or reused. Federal, state, and local laws establish regulations for the disposal of sharps containers. In some areas, the filled container is placed in a special oven and melted. The material remaining is packaged as biohazard or infectious waste

and disposed of according to legal requirements for infectious waste.

Spills or splashes of blood, body fluids, secretions, or excretions must be wiped up immediately (see figure 13-15). Gloves must be worn while wiping up the area with disposable cleaning cloths. The area must then be cleaned with a disinfectant solution such as a 10-percent bleach solution. Furniture or equipment contaminated by the spill or splash must be cleaned and disinfected immediately. For large spills, an

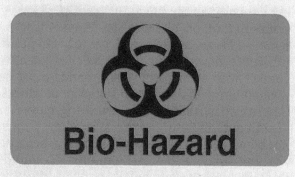

FIGURE 13-14 The universal biohazard symbol indicates a potential source of infection.

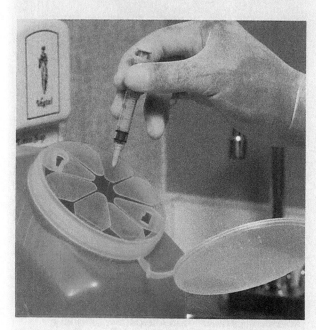

FIGURE 13-13 All needles and sharp objects must be discarded immediately in a leakproof puncture-resistant sharps container.

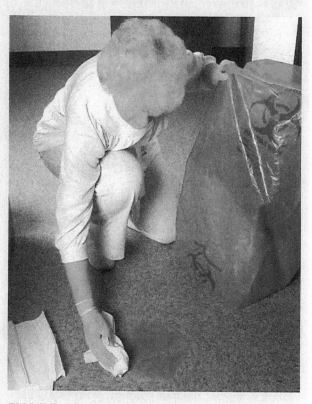

FIGURE 13-15 Gloves must be worn while wiping up any spills of blood, body fluids, secretions, or excretions.

absorbent powder may be used to soak up the fluid. After the fluid is absorbed, it is swept up and placed in an infectious waste container.

Whenever possible, mouthpieces or resuscitation devices should be used to avoid the need for mouth-to-mouth resuscitation. These devices should be placed in convenient locations and be readily accessible for use.

To dispose of waste and soiled linen, wear gloves and follow the agency policy developed according to law. Infectious wastes such as contaminated dressings; gloves; urinary drainage bags; incontinent pads; vaginal pads; disposable emesis basins, bedpans, and/or urinals; and body tissues must be placed in special infectious waste or biohazardous material bags (see figure 13-16) according to law. Other trash is frequently placed in plastic bags and incinerated. The health care worker must dispose of waste in the proper container (see figure 13-17) and know the requirements for disposal. Soiled linen should be placed in laundry bags to prevent any contamination. Linen soiled with blood, body fluids, or excretions is placed in a special bag for contaminated linen and is usually soaked in a disinfectant prior to being laundered. Gloves must be worn while handling any contaminated linen, and any bag containing contaminated linen must be clearly labeled and color coded.

Any cut, injury, needle stick, or splashing of blood or body fluids must be reported immediately. Agency policy must be followed to deal with the injury or contamination. Every health care facility must have a policy for documenting any exposure incident, recording the care given, noting follow-up to the exposure incident, and identifying ways to prevent a similar incident.

Standard precautions must be followed at all times by all health care workers. By observing these precautions, health care workers can help break the chain of infection and protect themselves, their patients, and all other individuals.

STUDENT: *Go to the workbook and complete the assignment sheet for 13:3, Observing Standard Precautions. Then return and continue with the procedure.*

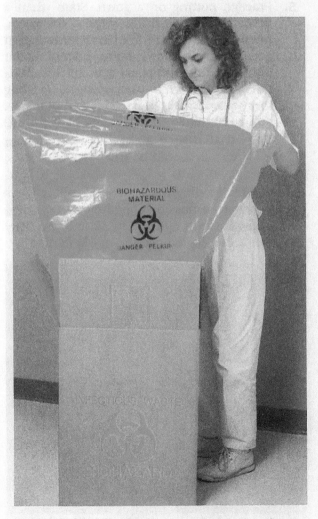

FIGURE 13-16 All infectious wastes must be placed in special infectious waste or biohazardous material bags.

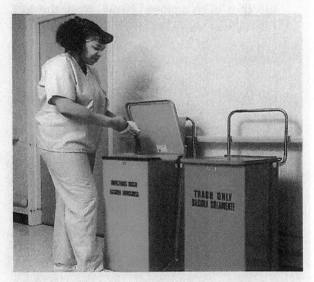

FIGURE 13-17 The health care worker must know the requirements for disposal of waste materials and dispose of wastes in the proper containers.

PROCEDURE 13:3
Observing Standard Precautions

Equipment and Supplies

Disposable gloves, infectious waste bags, needle and syringe, sharps container, gown, masks, protective eyewear, resuscitation devices

NOTE: This procedure will help you learn standard precautions. It is important for you to observe these precautions at all times while working in the laboratory or clinical area.

Procedure

1. Assemble equipment.
2. Review the precautions in the information section for Observing Standard Precautions. Note points that are not clear, and ask your instructor for an explanation.
3. Practice handwashing according to Procedure 13:2. Identify at least six times that hands must be washed according to standard precautions.
4. Name four instances when gloves must be worn to observe standard precautions. Put on a pair of disposable gloves. Practice removing the gloves without contaminating the skin. With a gloved hand, grasp the cuff of the glove on the opposite hand, handling only the outside of the glove (see figure 13-18A). Pull the glove down and turn it inside out while removing it. Take care not to touch the skin with the gloved hand. Using the ungloved hand, slip the fingers under the cuff of the glove on the opposite hand (see figure 13-18B). Touching only the inside of the glove and taking care not to touch the skin, pull the glove down and turn it inside out while removing it. Place the gloves in an infectious waste container. Wash your hands immediately.
5. Practice putting on a gown. State when a gown is to be worn. To remove the gown, touch only the inside. Fold the contaminated gown so the outside is folded inward. Roll it into a bundle and place it in an infectious waste container if it is disposable, or in a bag for contaminated linen if it is not disposable.

    CAUTION: If a gown is contaminated, gloves should be worn while removing the gown.

    NOTE: Folding the gown and rolling it prevents transmission of pathogens.

6. Practice putting on a mask and protective eyewear. To remove the mask, handle it by

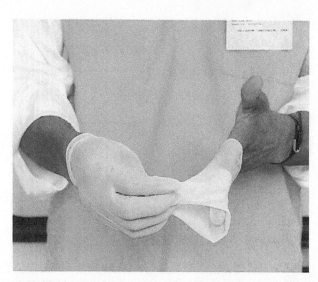

FIGURE 13-18A To remove the first glove, use a gloved hand to grasp the outside of the glove on the opposite hand. Pull the glove down and turn it inside out while removing it.

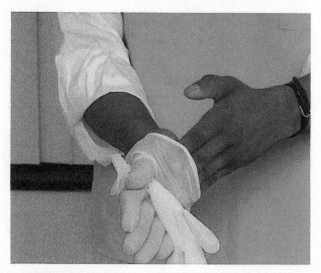

FIGURE 13-18B To remove the second glove, slip the fingers of the ungloved hand inside the cuff of the glove. Touch only the inside of the glove while pulling it down and turning it inside out.

the ties only. Clean and disinfect protective eyewear after use.

7. Practice proper disposal of sharps. Uncap a needle attached to a syringe, taking care not to stick yourself with the needle. Place the entire needle and syringe in a sharps container. State the rules regarding disposal of the sharps container.

8. Spill a small amount of water on a counter. Pretend that it is blood. Put on gloves and use disposable cloths or gauze to wipe up the spill. Put the contaminated cloths or gauze in an infectious waste bag. Use clean disposable cloths or gauze to wipe the area thoroughly with a disinfectant agent. Put the cloths or gauze in the infectious waste bag, remove your gloves, and wash your hands.

9. Practice handling an infectious waste bag. Fold down the top edge of the bag to form a cuff at the top of the bag. Wear gloves to close the bag after contaminated wastes have been placed in it. Put your hands under the folded cuff (see figure 13-19A) and gently expel excess air from the bag. Twist the top of the bag shut and fold down the top edges to seal the bag. Secure the fold with tape or a tie according to agency policy (see figure 13-19B).

10. Examine mouthpieces and resuscitation devices that can be used in place of mouth-to-mouth resuscitation. You will be taught to use these devices when you learn cardiopulmonary resuscitation (CPR).

11. Discuss the following situations with another student and determine which standard precautions should be observed:

   ◆ A patient has an open sore on the skin and pus is seeping from the area. You are going to bathe the patient.

   ◆ You are cleaning a tray of instruments that contains a disposable surgical blade and needle with syringe.

   ◆ A tube of blood drops to the floor and breaks, spilling the blood on the floor.

   ◆ Drainage from dressings on an infected wound has soiled the linen on the bed you are changing.

   ◆ You work in a dental office and are assisting a dentist while a tooth is being extracted (removed).

12. Replace all equipment used.

Practice *Go to the workbook and use the evaluation sheet for 13:3, Observing Standard Precautions. When you feel you have mastered this skill, sign the sheet and give it to your instructor for further action.*

 Final Checkpoint Using the criteria listed on the evaluation sheet, your instructor will grade your performance.

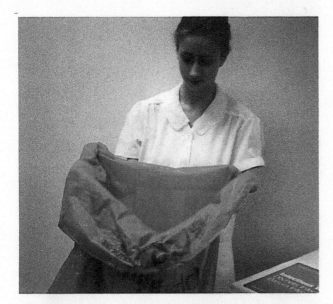

FIGURE 13-19A To close an infectious waste bag, wear gloves and place your hands under the cuff to gently expel excess air.

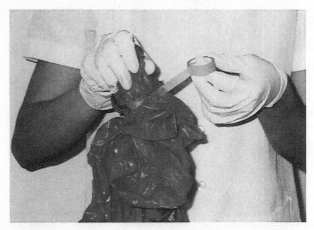

FIGURE 13-19B After folding down the top edge of the infectious waste bag, tie or tape it securely.

13:4 INFORMATION Sterilizing with an Autoclave

Sterilization of instruments and equipment is essential in preventing the spread of infection. In any of the health fields, you may be responsible for proper sterilization. The following basic principles relate to sterilization methods. The autoclave is the safest, most efficient sterilization method.

An **autoclave** is a piece of equipment that uses steam under pressure or gas to sterilize equipment and supplies (see figure 13-20). It is the most efficient method of sterilizing most articles, and it will destroy all microorganisms, both pathogenic and nonpathogenic, including spores and viruses.

Autoclaves are available in various sizes and types. Offices and health clinics usually have smaller units, and hospitals or surgical areas have large floor model units. A pressure cooker can be used in home situations.

Before any equipment or supplies are sterilized in an autoclave, they must be prepared properly. All items must be washed thoroughly and then rinsed. Oily substances can often be removed with alcohol or ether. Any residue left on articles will tend to bake and stick to the article during the autoclaving process.

Items that are to remain sterile must be wrapped before they are autoclaved. A wide variety of wraps are available. The wrap must be a material that will allow for the penetration of steam during the autoclaving process. Samples of wraps include muslin, autoclave paper, special plastic or paper bags, and autoclave containers (see figure 13-21).

Autoclave indicators are used to ensure that articles have been sterilized (see figure 13-22). Examples of indicators include autoclave tape, sensitivity marks on bags or wraps, and indicator capsules. The indicator is usually placed on or near the article when the article is put into the autoclave. Indicators can also be placed in the center of a package, such as a tray of instruments, to show that sterilization of the entire package has occurred. The indicator will change appearance during the autoclaving process because of time and temperature, which leads to sterilization. Learn how to recognize that an article is sterile by reading the directions provided with indicators.

The autoclave must be loaded correctly in order for all parts of an article to be sterilized. Steam builds at the top of the chamber and moves downward. As it moves down, it pushes cool, dry air out of the bottom of the chamber. Therefore, materials must be placed so the

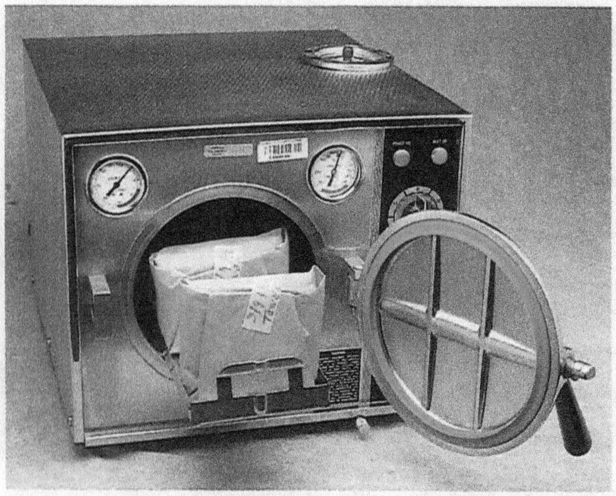

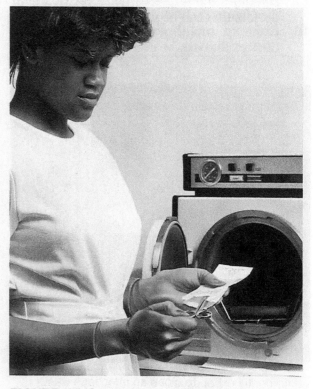

FIGURE 13-20 An autoclave uses steam under pressure to sterilize items.

FIGURE 13-21 Special plastic or paper autoclave bags can be used to sterilize instruments.

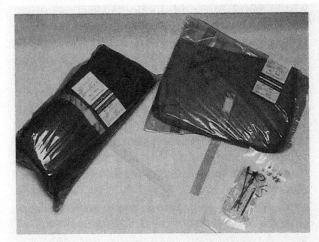

FIGURE 13-22 Autoclave indicators change color to show that sterilization has occurred. The strips below each package show how the indicators looked before sterilization.

steam can penetrate along the natural planes between the packages of articles in the autoclave. Place the articles in such a way that there is space between all pieces. Packages should be placed on the sides, not flat. Jars, basins, and cans should be placed on their sides, not flat, so that steam can enter and air can flow out. No articles should come in contact with the sides, top, or door of the autoclave.

The length of time and amount of pressure required to sterilize different items varies (see figure 13-23). *It is important to check the directions that come with the autoclave.* Because different types of articles require different times and pressures, it is important to separate loads so that all articles sterilized at one time require the same time and pressure. For example, rubber tubings usually require a relatively short period of time and can be damaged by long exposure. Certain instruments and needles require a longer period of time to ensure sterilization; so, items of this type should not be sterilized in the same load as are rubber tubings.

Wet surfaces permit rapid infiltration of organisms, so it is important that all items are thoroughly dry before being removed from the autoclave. The length of time for drying varies. Follow the manufacturer's instructions.

Sterilized items must be stored in clean, dustproof areas. Items usually remain sterile for 30 days after autoclaving. However, if the wraps loosen or tear, if they become wet, or if any chance of contamination occurs, the items should be rewrapped and autoclaved again.

ARTICLES	TIME AT 250° TO 254°F (121° TO 123°C)
Glassware: empty, inverted	15 minutes
Instruments: metal in covered or open, padded or unpadded tray	
Needles, unwrapped	
Syringes: unassembled, unwrapped	
Instruments, metal combined with other materials in covered and/or padded tray	
Instruments wrapped in double-thickness muslin	20 minutes
Flasked solutions, 75–250 mL	
Needles, individually packaged in glass tubes or paper	
Syringes: unassembled, individually packed in muslin or paper	30 minutes
Dressings wrapped in paper or muslin (small packs only)	
Flasked solutions, 500–1,000 mL	
Sutures: silk, cotton, or nylon; wrapped in paper or muslin	
Treatment trays wrapped in muslin or paper	

FIGURE 13-23 The length of time required to sterilize different items varies.

NOTE: At the end of the 30-day sterile period—providing that the wrap has not loosened, been torn, or gotten wet—remove the old autoclave tape from the package, replace with a new, dated tape, and resterilize according to correct procedure.

Some autoclaves are equipped with a special door that allows the autoclave to be used as a dry-heat sterilizer. Dry heat involves the use of a high temperature for a long period of time. The temperature is usually a minimum of 320°F to 350°F (160°C to 177°C). The minimum time is usually 60 minutes. Dry-heat sterilization is a good method for sterilizing instruments that may corrode, such as knife blades, or items that would be destroyed by the moisture in steam sterilization, such as powders. Dry heat should never be used on soft rubber goods because the heat will destroy the rubber. Some types of plastic will also melt in dry heat. An oven can be used for dry-heat sterilization in home situations.

Procedures 13:4A and 13:4B, following, describe wrapping articles for autoclaving and autoclaving techniques. These procedures vary in different agencies and areas, but the same principles apply. In some facilities, many supplies are purchased as sterile, disposable items; needles and syringes are purchased in sterilized wraps, used once, and then destroyed. In other facilities, however, special treatment trays are sterilized and used more than one time.

It is important that you follow the directions specific to the autoclave with which you are working, and the agency policy for sterile supplies. Careless autoclaving permits the transmission of disease-producing organisms. Infection control is everyone's responsibility.

STUDENT: *Go to the workbook and complete the assignment sheet for 13:4, Sterilizing with an Autoclave. Then return and continue with the procedures.*

PROCEDURE 13:4A
Wrapping Items for Autoclaving

Equipment and Supplies

Items to wrap: instrument, towel, bowl; autoclave wrap: paper, muslin, plastic or paper bag; autoclave tape or indicator; disposable or utility gloves; pen or autoclave marker; masking tape (if autoclave tape is not used)

Procedure

1. Assemble equipment.
2. Wash hands. Put on gloves.

    CAUTION: If the items to be autoclaved are contaminated with blood, body fluids, or tissues, gloves must be worn while cleaning the items.
3. Sanitize the items to be sterilized. Instruments, bowls, and similar items should be cleaned thoroughly in soapy water (see figure 13-24). Rinse the items well in cool water to remove any soapy residue. Then rinse well with hot water. Dry the items with a towel. After the items are sanitized and dry, remove the gloves and wash hands.

    NOTE: If stubborn stains are present, it may be necessary to soak the items.

    NOTE: Check the teeth on serrated (notched like a saw) instruments. Scrub with a brush as necessary.

4. To prepare linen for wrapping, check first to make sure it is clean and dry. Fold the linen in half lengthwise. If it is very wide, fold lengthwise again. Fanfold or accordion pleat the linen from end to end until a compact package is formed (see figure 13-25A). All folds should be the same size. Fold back

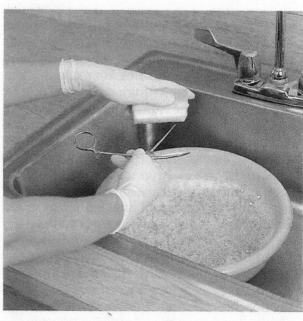

FIGURE 13-24 Wear gloves to scrub instruments thoroughly with soapy water.

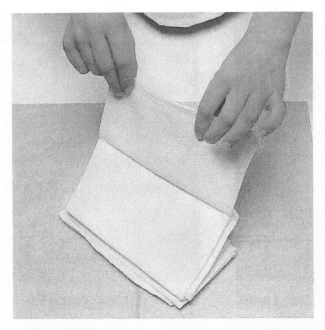

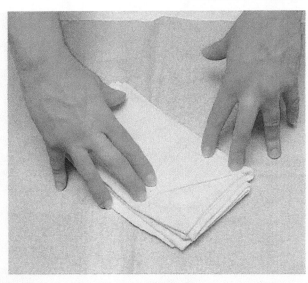

FIGURE 13-25B Fold back one corner on the top fold of the linen.

FIGURE 13-25A Fanfold clean, dry linen so all the folds are the same size.

one corner on the top fold (see figure 13-25B). This provides a piece to grab when opening the linen.

NOTE: Fanfolding linens allows for easy handling after sterilization.

5. Select the correct wrap for the item. Make sure the wrap is large enough to enclose the item to be wrapped.

NOTE: Double-thickness muslin, disposable paper wraps, and plastic or paper bags are the most common wraps.

6. With the wrap positioned at a diagonal angle and one corner pointing toward you, place the item to be sterilized in the center of the wrap.

NOTE: Make sure that hinged instruments are open so the steam can sterilize all edges.

7. Fold up the bottom corner to the center (see figure 13-26A). Double back a small corner (see figure 13-26B).

8. Fold a side corner over to the center. Make sure the edges are sealed and that there are no air pockets. Bring back a small corner (see figure 13-26C).

   ⚠ CAUTION: Any open areas at corners will allow pathogens to enter.

9. Fold in the other side corner. Again, watch for and avoid open edges. Bring back a small corner (see figure 13-26D).

10. Bring the final corner up and over the top of the package. Check the two edges to be sure they are sealed and tight. Tuck this under the pocket created by the previous folds. Leave a small corner exposed so it can be used when unwrapping the package (see figure 13-26E).

    NOTE: This is frequently called an "envelope" wrap, because the final corner is tucked into the wrap similar to the way the flap is tucked into an envelope.

11. Secure with autoclave or pressure-sensitive indicator tape.

    NOTE: If regular masking tape is used, attach an autoclave indicator to reflect when contents are sterilized.

12. Label the package by marking the tape with the date and contents (see figure 13-26F). Some health care agencies may require you to initial the label.

    NOTE: For certain items, the type or size of item should be noted, for example, curved hemostat or mosquito hemostat, hand towel or bath towel, small bowl or large bowl.

    NOTE: Contents will not be sterile after 30 days, so the date of sterilization must be noted on the package.

13. Check the package. It should be firm enough for handling but loose enough for proper circulation of steam.

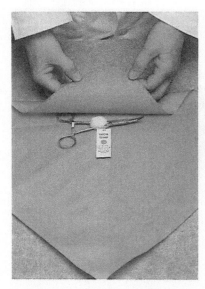

FIGURE 13-26A Place the instrument in the center of the wrap. Fold the bottom corner in to the center.

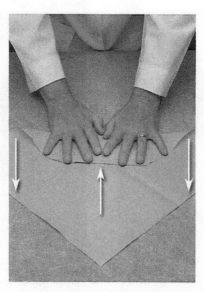

FIGURE 13-26B Turn a small corner back to form a tab.

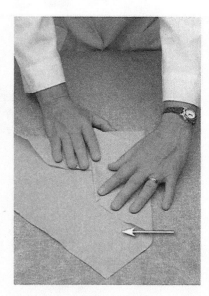

FIGURE 13-26C Fold in one side and fold back a tab.

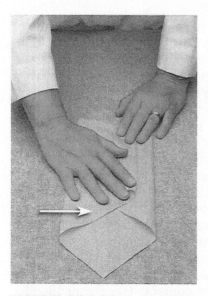

FIGURE 13-26D Fold in the opposite side and fold back a tab.

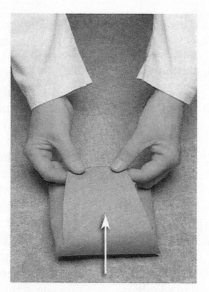

FIGURE 13-26E Bring the final corner up and over the top of the pack and tuck it in, leaving a small corner exposed.

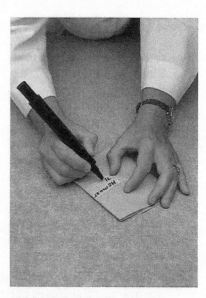

FIGURE 13-26F Secure the package with autoclave tape. Label it with the date, contents, and your initials.

14. To use a plastic or paper autoclave bag (refer to figure 13-21), select or cut the correct size for the item to be sterilized. Place the clean item inside the bag. Double fold the open end(s) and tape or secure with autoclave tape. Check the package to make sure it is secure.

NOTE: In some agencies, the ends are sealed with heat prior to autoclaving.

NOTE: If the bag has an autoclave indicator, regular masking tape can be used to seal the ends.

15. Replace all equipment used.

16. Wash hands.

Practice *Go to the workbook and use the evaluation sheet for 13:4A, Wrapping Items for Autoclaving, to practice this procedure. When you feel you have mastered this skill, sign the sheet and give it to your instructor for further action.*

 Final Checkpoint Using the criteria listed on the evaluation sheet, your instructor will grade your performance.

PROCEDURE 13:4B

Loading and Operating an Autoclave

NOTE: Follow the operating instructions for your autoclave. The basic principles of loading apply to all autoclaves. Basic controls for one autoclave are shown in figure 13-27.

Equipment and Supplies

Autoclave, distilled water, small pitcher or measuring cup, items wrapped or prepared for autoclaving, time chart for autoclave, 13:4 Information section

Procedure

Review the Information section for 13:4, Sterilizing with an Autoclave. Then proceed with the following activities. You should read through the

procedure first, checking against the diagram. Then practice with an autoclave.

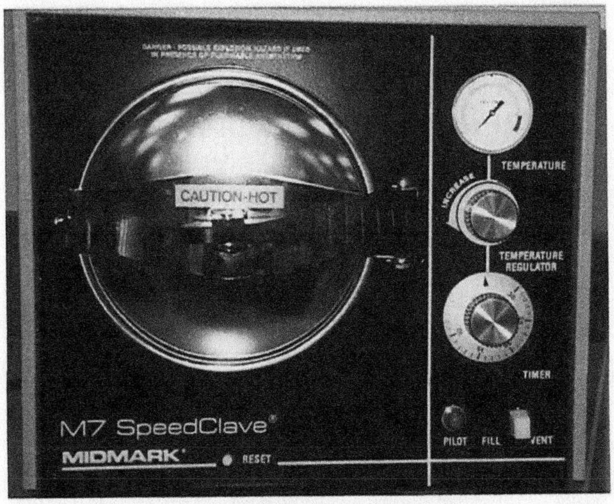

1. Assemble equipment.
2. Wash and dry hands thoroughly.
3. Check the three-prong plug and the electrical cord. If either is damaged or prongs are missing, do not use the autoclave. If no problems are present, plug the cord into a wall outlet.
4. Use distilled water to fill the reservoir to within 2 1/2 inches below the opening or to the level indicated on the autoclave.
   NOTE: Distilled water prevents the collection of mineral deposits and prolongs the life and effectiveness of the autoclave.
5. Check the pressure gauge to make sure it is at zero.
   CAUTION: Never open the door unless the pressure is zero.
6. Open the safety door by following the manufacturer's instructions. Some door handles require an upward and inward pressure; others require a side-pressure technique.
7. Load the autoclave. Make sure all articles have been prepared correctly. Check for autoclave indicators, secure wraps, and correct labels. Separate loads so all items require the same time, temperature, and pressure. Place packages on their sides. Place bowls or basins on their sides so air and steam can flow in and out of the container (see figure 13-28). Make sure there is space between the packages so the steam can circulate.
   NOTE: Check to make sure no large packages block the steam flow to smaller packages. Place large packages on the bottom.

FIGURE 13-27 Autoclave control valves vary, but most contain the same basic controls.

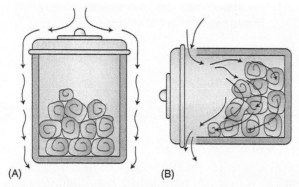

(A)   (B)

FIGURE 13-28 Bowls or basins should be placed on their sides in the autoclave so air and steam can flow in and out of the container: **(A)** shows incorrect placement, while **(B)** shows correct placement.

CAUTION: Make sure no item comes in contact with the sides, top, or door of the autoclave chamber.

8. Follow the instructions for filling the chamber with the correct amount of water. Most autoclaves have a "Fill" setting on the control. Allow water to enter the chamber until the water covers the fill plate inside the chamber.

9. When the correct amount of water is in the chamber, follow the instructions for stopping the flow of water. In many autoclaves, turning the control valve to "Sterilize" stops the flow of water from the reservoir.

10. Check the load in the chamber to be sure it is properly spaced. The chamber can also be loaded at this point, if this has not been done previously.

11. Close and lock the door.

    CAUTION: Be sure the door is securely locked; check by pulling slightly.

12. Read the time chart for the specific time and temperature required for sterilization of items that were placed in the autoclave.

13. After referring to the chart provided with the autoclave or reviewing figure 13-23, set the control valves to allow the temperature and pressure to increase in the autoclave.

14. When the desired temperature (usually 250° to 255°F or 121° to 123°C) and pressure (usually 15 pounds) have been reached, set the controls to maintain the desired temperature during the sterilization process. Follow the manufacturer's instructions.

15. Based on the information in the time chart, set the timer to the correct time.

NOTE: Many autoclaves require you to rotate the timer past 10 (minutes) before setting the time.

16. Check the pressure and temperature gauges at intervals to make sure they remain as originally set.

    NOTE: Most autoclaves automatically shut off when pressure reaches 35 pounds.

17. When the required time has passed, set the controls so the autoclave will vent the steam from the chamber.

18. Put on safety glasses.

    CAUTION: *Never* open the door without glasses. The escaping steam can burn the eyes.

19. Check the pressure and temperature gauges. When the pressure gauge is at zero, and the temperature gauge is at or below 212°F, open the door about 1/2 to 1 inch to permit thorough drying of contents.

    CAUTION: Do not open the door until pressure is zero.

20. After the autoclaved items are dry, remove and store them in a dry, dust-free area.

    CAUTION: Handle supplies and equipment carefully. They may be hot.

21. If there are additional loads to run, leave the main valve in the vent position. This will keep the autoclave ready for immediate use.

22. If this is the final load, turn the autoclave off. Unplug the cord from the wall outlet; do not pull on the cord.

    NOTE: The autoclave must be cleaned on a regular basis. Follow manufacturer's instructions.

23. Replace all equipment used.

24. Wash hands.

Practice *Go to the workbook and use the evaluation sheet for 13:4B, Loading and Operating an Autoclave, to practice this procedure. When you feel you have mastered this skill, sign the sheet and give it to your instructor for further action.*

 Final Checkpoint Using the criteria listed on the evaluation sheet, your instructor will grade your performance.

13:5 INFORMATION Using Chemicals for Disinfection

Many health fields require the use of chemicals for aseptic control. Certain points that must be observed while using the chemicals are discussed in the following information.

Chemicals are frequently used for aseptic control. Many chemicals do not kill spores and viruses; therefore, chemicals are not a method of sterilization. Because sterilization does not occur, **chemical disinfection** is the appropriate term (rather than cold sterilization, a term sometimes used). A few chemicals will kill spores and viruses, but these chemicals frequently require that instruments be submerged in the chemical for ten or more hours. It is essential to read an entire label to determine the effectiveness of the product before using any chemical.

Chemicals are used to disinfect instruments that do not penetrate body tissue. Many dental instruments, percussion hammers, scissors, and similar items are examples. In addition, chemicals are used to disinfect thermometers and other items that would be destroyed by the high heat used in the autoclave.

Proper cleaning of all instruments or articles is essential. Particles or debris on items may contaminate the chemicals and reduce their effectiveness. In addition, all items must be rinsed thoroughly because the presence of soap can also reduce the effectiveness of chemicals. The articles must be dry before being placed in the disinfectant in order to keep the chemical at its most effective strength.

Some chemical solutions used as disinfectants are 90-percent isopropyl alcohol, formaldehyde–alcohol, 2-percent phenolic germicide, 10-percent bleach (sodium hypochlorite) solution, glutaraldehyde, iodophor, Lysol, Cidex, and benzalkonium (zephiran). The manufacturer's directions should be read completely before using any solution. Some solutions must be diluted or mixed before use. The directions will also specify the recommended time for the most thorough disinfection.

Chemical solutions can cause rust to form on certain instruments, so antirust tablets or solutions are frequently added to the chemicals. Again, it is important to read the directions provided with the tablets or solution. If improperly used, antirust substances may cause a chemical reaction with a solution and reduce the effectiveness of the chemical disinfectant.

The container used for chemical disinfection must be large enough to accommodate the items. In addition, the items should be separate so each one will come in contact with the chemical. A tight-fitting lid must be placed on the container while the articles are in the solution.

The chemical disinfectant must completely cover the article. This is the only way to be sure that all parts of the article will be disinfected.

Before removing items from solutions, health workers must wash their hands. Sterile pick-ups or transfer forceps may be used to remove the instruments from the solution. The instruments are placed on a sterile or clean towel to dry, and then stored in a drawer or dust-free closet.

Solutions must be changed frequently. Some solutions can be used over a period of time, but others must be discarded after one use. Follow the manufacturer's instructions. However, any time contamination occurs or dirt is present in the solution, discard it. A fresh solution must be used.

STUDENT: *Go to the Workbook and complete the assignment sheet for 13:5, Using Chemicals for disinfection. Then return and continue with the procedure.*

PROCEDURE 13:5
Using Chemicals for Disinfection

Equipment and Supplies

Chemicals, container with tight-fitting lid, basin, soap, water, instruments, brush, sterile pick-ups or transfer forceps, sterile towel, disposable gloves

Procedure

1. Assemble equipment.
2. Wash hands. Put on gloves.

    NOTE: Wear gloves if any of the instruments or equipment are contaminated with blood or body fluids.

3. Wash all instruments or equipment thoroughly. Use warm soapy water. Use the brush on serrated edges of instruments.
4. Rinse in cool water to remove soapy residue. Then rinse well with hot water. Dry all instruments or equipment thoroughly.

    NOTE: Water on the instruments or equipment will dilute the chemical disinfectant.

5. Check container. Make sure lid fits securely.

    NOTE: A loose cover will permit entrance of pathogens.

6. Place instruments in the container. Make sure there is a space between instruments. Leave hinged edges open so the solution can flow between the surfaces.
7. Carefully read label instructions about the chemical solution. Some solutions must be diluted. Check the manufacturer's recommended soaking time.

    CAUTION: Reread instructions to be sure solution is safe to use on instruments.

    NOTE: An antirust substance must be added to some solutions.

8. Pour solution into the container slowly to avoid splashing. Make sure that all instruments are covered (see figure 13-29). Close the lid of the container.

    NOTE: Read label three times: before pouring, while pouring, and after pouring.

    CAUTION: Avoid splashing the chemical on your skin. Improper handling of chemicals may cause burns and/or injuries.

9. Remove gloves. Wash hands.
10. Leave the instruments in the solution for the length of time recommended by the manufacturer.

    NOTE: Twenty to thirty minutes is the usual soaking time.

11. When instruments have soaked the correct amount of time, use sterile pick-ups or transfer forceps to remove the instruments from the solution. Place them on a sterile towel to dry. A second sterile towel is sometimes used to cover the instruments while they are drying. Store the instruments in special drawers, containers, or dust-free closets.

    NOTE: Some contamination occurs when instruments are exposed to the air. In some cases, such as with external instruments, this minimal contamination will not affect usage.

12. Replace all equipment used.

    CAUTION: If the disinfectant solution can be used again, label the container with the name of the disinfectant, date, and number of days it can be used according to manufacturer's instructions. When solutions cannot be reused, dispose of the solution according to manufacturer's instructions.

13. Wash hands.

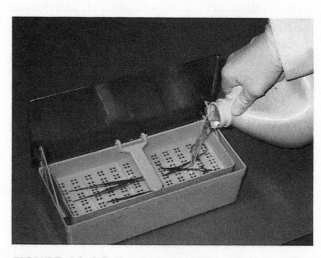

FIGURE 13-29 Pour the chemical disinfectant into the container until all instruments are covered with solution.

Practice *Go to the workbook and use the evaluation sheet for 13:5, Using Chemicals for Disinfection, to practice this procedure. When you feel you have mastered this skill, sign the sheet and give it to your instructor for further action.*

Final Checkpoint Using the criteria listed on the evaluation sheet, your instructor will grade your performance.

13:6 INFORMATION Cleaning with an Ultrasonic Unit

Ultrasonic units are used in many dental and medical offices and other health agencies to clean a large variety of instruments prior to sterilizing them. The following information explains operation of the unit.

Ultrasonic cleaning is used on a large variety of instruments and items in health care agencies. An ultrasonic unit uses sound waves to clean. When the unit is turned on, the sound waves produce millions of microscopic bubbles in a cleaning solution. When the bubbles strike the items being cleaned, they explode, a process known as **cavitation,** and drive the cleaning solution onto the article. Accumulated dirt and residue are easily and gently removed from the article.

Ultrasonic cleaning is not sterilization because spores and viruses remain on the articles. If sterilization is desired, other methods must be used after the ultrasonic cleaning.

Only ultrasonic solutions should be used in the unit. Different solutions are available for different materials. A general, all-purpose cleaning solution is usually used in the permanent tank and to clean many items. There are other specific solutions for alginate, plaster and stone removal, and tartar removal. The solution chart provided with the ultrasonic unit will state which solution should be used. It is important to read labels carefully before using any solutions. Some solutions must be diluted before use. Some can be used only on specific materials. All solutions are toxic. They can also

cause skin irritation, so contact with the skin and eyes should be avoided. Solutions should be discarded when they become cloudy or contaminated, or if cleaning results are poor.

The permanent tank of the ultrasonic unit (figure 13-30) must contain a solution at all times. A general, all-purpose cleaning solution is used most of the time. Glass beakers or auxiliary pans or baskets can then be placed in the permanent tank. The items to be cleaned and the proper

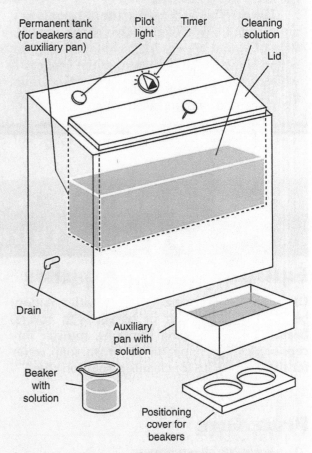

FIGURE 13-30 Parts of an ultrasonic cleaning unit.

cleaning solution are then put in the beakers or pans. The bottoms of the beakers or pans must always be positioned below the level of the solution present in the permanent tank. In this way, cavitation can be transmitted from the main tank and through the solution to the items being cleaned in the beakers or pans. Never run the ultrasonic unit unless solutions are in both containers. In addition, the items being cleaned must be submerged in the cleaning solution.

Many different items can be cleaned in an ultrasonic unit. Examples include instruments, impression trays, glass products, and most jewelry. Do not use the ultrasonic unit on jewelry with pearls or pasted stones. The sound waves can destroy the pearls or the paste holding the stones. Prior to cleaning, most of the dirt or particles should be brushed off the items being cleaned. It is better to clean a few articles at a time and avoid overloading the unit. If items are close together, the process of cavitation is poor because the bubbles cannot strike all parts of the items being cleaned.

The glass beakers used in the ultrasonic unit are made of a type of glass that allows the passage of sound waves. After continual use, the sound waves etch the bottom of the beakers. A white, opaque coating forms. The beakers must be discarded and replaced when this occurs.

After each use, the beakers should be washed with soap and water and rinsed thoroughly to remove any soapy residue. They must be dry before being filled with solution because water in the beaker can dilute the solution.

The permanent tank of the unit must be drained and cleaned at intervals based on tank use or appearance of the solution in the tank. A drain valve on the side of the tank is opened to allow the solution to drain. The tank is then wiped with a damp cloth or disinfectant. Another damp cloth or disinfectant is used to wipe off the outside of the unit. Never submerge the unit in water to clean it. After cleaning, a fresh solution should be placed in the permanent tank.

Read the manufacturer's instructions carefully before using any ultrasonic unit. Most manufacturers provide cleaning charts that state the type of solution and time required for a variety of cleaning problems. Each time an item is cleaned in an ultrasonic unit, the chart should be used to determine the correct cleaning solution and time required.

STUDENT: *Go to the workbook and complete the assignment sheet for 13:6, Cleaning with an Ultrasonic Unit. Then return and continue with the procedure.*

PROCEDURE 13:6

Cleaning with an Ultrasonic Unit

Equipment and Supplies

Ultrasonic unit, permanent tank with solution, beakers, auxiliary pan or basket with covers, beaker bands, cleaning solutions, transfer forceps or pick-ups, paper towels, brush, soap, water for rinsing, articles for cleaning, solution chart

Procedure

1. Assemble all equipment.
2. Wash hands. Put on gloves if any items are contaminated with blood, body fluids, secretions, or excretions.

3. Use a brush and soap and water to remove any large particles of dirt from articles to be cleaned. Rinse articles thoroughly. Dry items.
   NOTE: Rinsing is important because soap may interact with the cleaning solution.
4. Check the permanent tank to be sure it has enough cleaning solution. An all-purpose cleaning solution is usually used in this tank.
   ! CAUTION: Never run the unit without solution in the permanent tank.
   NOTE: Many solutions must be diluted before use; if new solution is needed, read the instructions on the bottle.

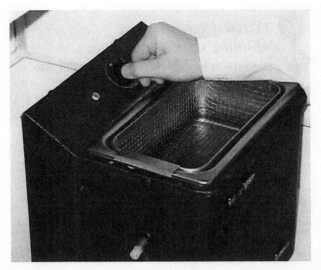

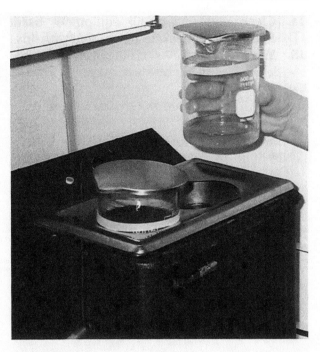

FIGURE 13-31 ABOVE The auxiliary basket can be used to clean larger items in an ultrasonic unit.
FIGURE 13-31 RIGHT Glass beakers can be used to clean smaller items in an ultrasonic unit.

5. Pour the proper cleaning solution into the auxiliary pan or beakers.
   NOTE: Use the cleaning chart to determine which solution to use.
   ! CAUTION: Read label before using.
   ! CAUTION: Handle solutions carefully. Avoid contact with skin and eyes.

6. Place the beakers, basket, or auxiliary pan into the permanent tank (see figure 13-31). Use beaker positioning covers and beaker bands. Beaker bands are large bands that circle the beakers to hold them in position and keep them from hitting the bottom of the permanent tank.

7. Check to be sure that the bottoms of the beakers, basket, or pan are below the level of solution in the permanent tank.
   NOTE: In order for sonic waves to flow through solutions in beakers, basket, or pan, the two solution levels must overlap.

8. Place articles to be cleaned in the beakers, basket, or pan. Be sure the solution completely covers the articles. Do not get solution on your hands.
   NOTE: Remember that pearls or pasted stones cannot be cleaned in an ultrasonic unit.

9. Turn the timer past 5 (minutes) and then set the proper cleaning time. Use the cleaning chart to determine the correct amount of time required for the items. Most articles are cleaned in 2 to 5 minutes.

10. Check that the unit is working. You should see a series of bubbles in both solutions. This is called cavitation.
    ! CAUTION: Do not get too close. Solution can spray into your face and eyes. Use beaker lids to prevent spray.

11. When the timer stops, cleaning is complete. Use transfer forceps or pick-ups to lift articles from the basket, pan, or beakers. Place the articles on paper towels. Then rinse articles thoroughly under running water.
    ! CAUTION: Avoid contact with skin. Solutions are toxic.

12. Allow articles to air dry or dry them with paper towels. Inspect the articles for cleanliness. If they are not clean, repeat the process.

13. Periodically change solutions in the permanent tank and auxiliary containers. Do this when solutions become cloudy or cleaning has not been effective. To clean the permanent tank, place a container under the side drain to collect the solution. Then open the valve and drain solution from the tank. Wash the inside with a damp cloth or disinfectant. To clean the auxiliary pans or beakers, discard the solution. (It can be poured down the sink, but allow water to run for a time after disposing of the solution.) Then wash the containers and rinse thoroughly.
    NOTE: If the bottoms of beakers are etched and white, the beakers must be discarded and replaced.

14. Clean and replace all equipment used. Make sure all beakers are covered with lids.
15. Wash hands.

Practice *Go to the workbook and use the evaluation sheet for 13:6, Cleaning with an Ultrasonic Unit, to practice this procedure. When you feel you have mastered this skill, sign the sheet and give it to your instructor for further action.*

 Final Checkpoint Using the criteria listed on the evaluation sheet, your instructor will grade your performance.

13:7 INFORMATION Using Sterile Techniques

Many procedures require the use of sterile techniques to protect the patient from further infection. *Surgical asepsis* refers to procedures that keep an object or area free from living organisms. The main facts are presented here.

Sterile means "free from all organisms," including spores and viruses. **Contaminated** means that organisms and pathogens are present. While working with sterile supplies, it is important that correct techniques be followed to maintain sterility and avoid contamination. It is also important that you are able to recognize sterile surfaces and contaminated surfaces.

A clean, uncluttered working area is required when working with sterile supplies. If other objects are in the way, it is easy to contaminate sterile articles. If sterile articles touch the skin or any part of your clothing, they are no longer sterile. Because any area below the waist is considered contaminated, sterile articles must be held away from and in front of the body and above the waist.

Once a **sterile field** has been set up (for example, a sterile towel has been placed on a tray), never reach across the top of the field. Microorganisms can drop from your arm or clothing and contaminate the field. Always reach in from either side to place additional articles on the field. Never turn your back to a sterile field.

The 2-inch border around the sterile field (towel-covered tray) is considered contaminated. Therefore, 2 inches around the outside of the field must not be used when sterile articles are placed on the sterile field.

Various techniques can be used to remove articles from sterile wraps, depending on the article being unwrapped. Some common techniques are the drop, mitten, and transfer-forceps techniques:

- *Drop technique:* for gauze pads, dressings, small items. The wrapper is partially opened and then held upside down over the sterile field. The item drops out of the wrapper and onto the sterile field (see figure 13-32A). It is important to keep fingers back so the article does not touch the skin as it falls out of the wrapper. It is also important to avoid touching the inside of the wrapper.

- *Mitten technique:* for bowls, drapes, linen, and other similar items. The wrapper is opened and its loose ends are grasped around the wrist with the opposite hand (see figure 13-32B). In this way, a mitten is formed around the hand that is still holding the item (for example, a bowl). With the mitten hand, the item can be placed on the sterile tray.

- *Transfer forceps:* for cotton balls, small items, or articles that cannot be removed by the drop or mitten techniques. Either sterile gloves or sterile transfer forceps (pick-ups) are used. Sterile transfer forceps or pick-ups are removed from their container of disinfectant solution and used to grasp the article from the opened package. Remove the item from the

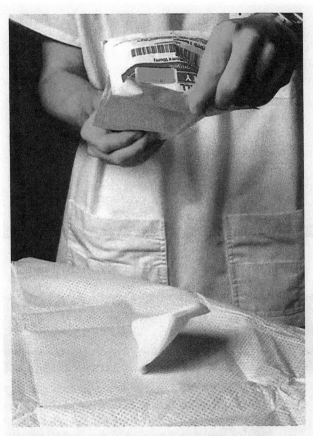

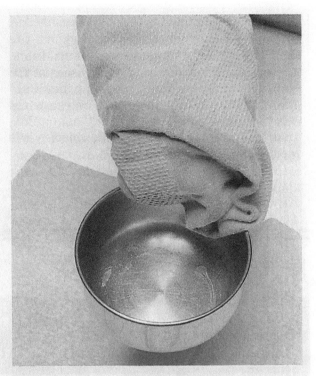

FIGURE 13-32B By using the wrap as a mitten, sterile supplies can be placed on a sterile field.

FIGURE 13-32A Sterile items can be dropped from the wrapper onto the sterile field.

opened, sterile wrap and place it on the sterile field (see figure 13-32C). It is important to keep the transfer forceps pointed in a downward direction. If they are pointed upward, the solution will flow back to the handle, become contaminated, and return to contaminate the sterile tips when they are being used to pick up items. In addition, care must be taken not to touch the sides or rim of the forceps container while removing or inserting the transfer forceps. Also, before using the transfer forceps, carefully shake them to get rid of excess disinfectant solution.

Organisms and pathogens travel quickly through a wet surface, so the sterile field must be kept dry. If a sterile towel or article gets wet, contamination has occurred. It is very important to use care when pouring solutions into sterile bowls or using solutions around a sterile field.

Make sure your sterile tray is open and you are ready to do the sterile procedure *before* putting the sterile gloves on your hands. Sterile

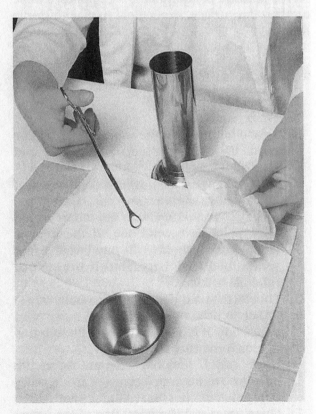

FIGURE 13-32C Sterile transfer forceps or pickups can be used to grasp sterile items and place them on a sterile field.

gloves are considered sterile on the outside and contaminated on the inside (side against the skin). Once they have been placed on the hands, it is important to hold the hands away from the body and above the waist to avoid contamination. You must handle only sterile objects while wearing sterile gloves.

If at any time during a procedure there is any suspicion that you have contaminated any article, start over. Never take a chance on using contaminated equipment or supplies.

A wide variety of commercially prepared sterile supplies is available. Packaged units are often set up for special procedures, such as changing dressings. Many agencies use these units instead of setting up special trays. Observe all sterile principles while using these units and read any directions provided with the units.

STUDENT: *Go to the workbook and complete the assignment sheet for 13:7, Using Sterile Techniques. Then return and continue with the procedures.*

PROCEDURE 13:7A
Opening Sterile Packages

Equipment and Supplies

Sterile package of equipment or supplies, a table or other flat surface, sterile field (tray with sterile towel)

Procedures

1. Assemble equipment.
2. Wash hands.
3. Take equipment to the area where it will be used. Check the autoclave indicator and date on the package.
   NOTE: Contents are not considered sterile if 30 days have elapsed since autoclaving.
4. Pick up the package with the tab or sealed edge pointing toward you. If the item is small, it can be held in the hand while being unwrapped. If it is large, place it on a table or other flat surface.
5. Loosen the wrapper fastener (usually tape).
6. Check to be sure the package is away from your body. If it is on a table, make sure it is not close to other objects.
   NOTE: Avoid possible contamination by keeping sterile supplies away from other objects.
7. Open the distal (furthest) flap of the wrapper by grasping the outside of the wrapper and pulling it away from you (see figure 13-33A).

⚠ **CAUTION:** Do not reach across the top of the package. Reach around the package to open it.

8. With one hand, raise a side flap and pull laterally (sideways) away from the package (see figure 13-33B).

⚠ **CAUTION:** Do *not* touch the inside of the wrapper at any time.

9. With the opposite hand, open the other side flap by pulling the tab to the side (see figure 13-33C).
   NOTE: Always reach in from the side. Never reach across the top of the sterile field or across any opened edges.

10. Open the proximal (closest) flap by lifting the flap up and toward you. Then drop it over the front of your hand (or the table) (see figure 13-33D).

⚠ **CAUTION:** Be careful not to touch the inside of the package or the contents of the package.

11. Transfer the contents of the sterile package using one of the following techniques:
    a. Drop: Separate the ends of the wrap and pull apart gently (see figure 13-34). Avoid touching the inside of the wrap. Secure the loose ends of the wrap and hold the package upside down over the sterile field. Allow the contents to drop onto the sterile tray.

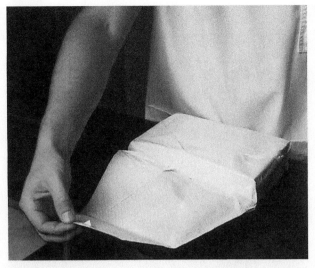

FIGURE 13-33A To open a sterile package, open the top flap away from you, handling only the outside of the wrap.

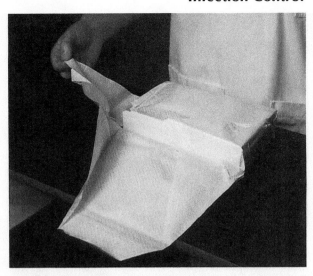

FIGURE 13-33B Open one side by pulling the wrap out to the side.

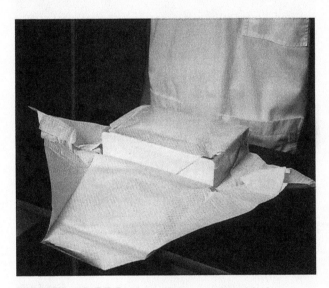

FIGURE 13-33C Open the opposite side by pulling the wrap out to the opposite side.

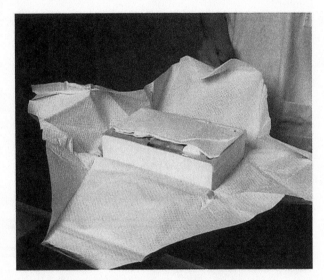

FIGURE 13-33D Open the side nearest to you by pulling back on the wrap.

b. Mitten: Grasp the contents securely by holding on to the outside of the wrapper as you unwrap it. With your free hand, gather the loose edges of the wrapper together and hold them securely around your wrist. This can be compared to making a mitten of the wrapper (with the sterile equipment on the outside of the mitten). Place the item on the sterile tray or hand it to someone who is wearing sterile gloves (refer to figure 13-32B).

c. Transfer forceps: Remove forceps from their sterile container, taking care not to touch the side or rim of the container with the forceps (see figure 13-35). Hold the forceps pointed downward. Shake them to remove excess disinfectant solution. Take care not to touch anything with the forceps. Use the forceps to grasp the item in the package and then place the item on the sterile tray.

NOTE: The method of transfer depends on the sterile item being transferred.

NOTE: If at any time during the procedure there is any suspicion that you have contaminated any article, start over. Never take a chance on using equipment for a sterile

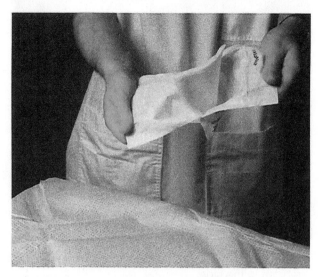

FIGURE 13-34 Separate the ends of the wrap and pull the edges apart gently without touching the contents.

procedure if there is any possibility that the equipment is contaminated.
12. Replace all equipment used.
13. Wash hands.

Practice *Go to the workbook and use the evaluation sheet for 13:7A, Opening Sterile Packages, to practice this procedure. When you feel you have mastered this skill, sign the sheet and give it to your instructor for further action.*

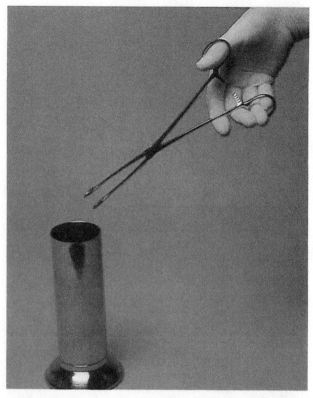

FIGURE 13-35 Remove the transfer or pick-up forceps without touching the sides or rim of the container and point them in a downward direction.

 Final Checkpoint Using the criteria listed on the evaluation sheet, your instructor will grade your performance.

PROCEDURE 13:7B

Preparing a Sterile Dressing Tray

Equipment and Supplies

Tray, sterile towels, sterile basin, sterile cotton balls or gauze sponges, sterile dressings (different sizes), antiseptic solution, forceps in disinfectant solution

Procedure

1. Assemble all equipment.
2. Wash hands.

3. Check the date and autoclave indicator for sterility. If more than 30 days have elapsed, use another package with a more recent date. Put the unsterile package aside for resterilization.
4. Place the tray on a flat surface or a Mayo stand.
   NOTE: Make sure the work area is clean and dry and there is sufficient room to work.
5. Open the package that contains the sterile towel. Be sure it is held away from your

body. Place the wrapper on a surface away from the tray or work area. Touch only the outside of the towel. Pick up the towel at its outer edge. Allow it to open by releasing the fanfolds. Place the towel with the outer side (side you have touched) on the tray. The untouched, or sterile, side will be facing up. Holding onto the outside edges of the towel, fanfold the back of the towel so the towel can be used later to cover the supplies.

CAUTION: Do not reach across the top of the towel. Reach in from either side.

NOTE: If you are setting up a relatively large work area, one towel may not be large enough when fanfolded to cover the supplies. In such a case, you will need a second sterile towel (later) to cover your sterile field.

CAUTION: At all times, make sure that you do *not* touch the sterile side of the towel. Avoid letting the towel come in contact with your uniform, other objects, or contaminated areas.

6. Correctly unwrap the package containing the sterile basin. Place the basin on the tray. Do not place it close to the edge of the towel.

NOTE: A 2-inch border around the outside edges of the towel is considered to be contaminated. No equipment should come in contact with this border.

CAUTION: Make sure that the wrapper does *not* touch the towel while placing the basin in position.

7. Unwrap the package containing the sterile cotton balls or gauze sponges. Use a dropping motion to place them in the basin. Do not touch the basin with the wrapper.

8. Unwrap the package containing the larger dressing. Use the sterile forceps to remove the dressing from the package and place it on the tray. Make sure the dressing is not too close to the edge of the towel.

NOTE: The larger, outside dressing is placed on the tray first (before other dressings). In this way, the supplies will be in the order of use. For example, gauze dressings placed directly on the skin will be on top of the pile, and a thick abdominal pad used on top of the gauze pads will be on the bottom of the pile.

NOTE: The forceps must be lifted straight up out of the container and must *not* touch the side or rim of the container. Keep the tips pointed down and above the waist at all times. Shake off excess disinfectant solution.

9. Unwrap the inner dressings correctly. Use the sterile forceps to place them on top of the other dressings on the sterile towel, or use a drop technique.

NOTE: Dressings are now in a pile; the dressing that will be used first is on the top of the pile.

NOTE: The number and type of dressings needed is determined by checking the patient being treated.

10. Open the bottle containing the correct antiseptic solution. Place the cap on the table, with the inside of the cap facing up. Pour a small amount of the solution into the sink to clean the lip of the bottle. Then hold the bottle over the basin and pour a sufficient amount of solution into the basin (see figure 13-36).

CAUTION: Make sure that no part of the bottle touches the basin or the sterile tray. Pour carefully to avoid splashing. If the tray gets wet, the entire tray will be contaminated, and you must begin again.

11. Check the tray to make sure all needed equipment is on it.

12. Pick up the fanfolded edge of the towel by placing one hand on each side edge of the towel on the underside, or contaminated side. Do not touch the sterile side. Keep your hands and arms to the side of the tray, and bring the towel forward to cover the supplies.

NOTE: A second sterile towel may be used to cover the supplies if the table or sterile field

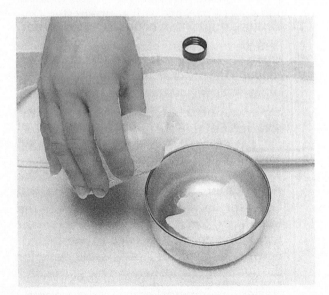

FIGURE 13-36 Avoid splashing the solution onto the sterile field while pouring it into the basin.

area is too large to be covered by the one fanfolded towel.

> **! CAUTION:** Never reach across the top of the sterile tray.

13. Once the sterile tray is ready, never allow it out of your sight. Take it to the patient area and use it immediately. If you need more equipment, you must take the tray with you. This is the only way to be completely positive that the tray does not become contaminated.
14. Replace equipment.
15. Wash hands.

Practice *Go to the workbook and use the evaluation sheet for 13:7B, Preparing a Sterile Dressing Tray, to practice this procedure. When you feel you have mastered this skill, sign the sheet and give it to your instructor for further action.*

 Final Checkpoint Using the criteria listed on the evaluation sheet, your instructor will grade your performance.

PROCEDURE 13:7C

Donning and Removing Sterile Gloves

Equipment and Supplies

Sterile gloves

Procedure

1. Assemble equipment and take it to the area where it is to be used. Check the date and/or autoclave indicator on the package to be sure gloves are still sterile. If they are not, put the package aside for re-sterilization and select a package with a current sterilization date.
2. Remove rings. Wash hands. Dry hands thoroughly.
3. Open the package of gloves, taking care not to touch the inside of the inner wrapper. The inner wrapper contains the gloves. Gently open it. The folded cuffs will be nearest you.

> **! CAUTION:** If you touch the *inside* of the package (where the gloves are), get a new package and start again.

4. The glove for the right hand will be on the right side and the glove for the left hand will be on the left side of the package. With the thumb and forefinger of the nondominant hand pick up the top edge of the folded-down cuff (inside of glove) of the glove for the dominant hand. Remove the glove carefully (see figure 13-37A).

> **! CAUTION:** Do *not* touch the outside of the glove. This is sterile. Only the part

that will be next to the skin can be touched. Remember, unsterile touches unsterile and sterile touches sterile.

5. Hold the glove by the inside cuff and slip the fingers and thumb of your other hand into the glove. Pull it on carefully (see figure 13-37B).

> **NOTE:** Hold the glove away from the body. Pull gently to avoid tearing the glove.

6. Insert your gloved hand under the cuff (outside) of the other glove and lift the glove from the package (see figure 13-37C). Do not touch any other area with your gloved hand while removing the glove from the package.

> **! CAUTION:** If contamination occurs, discard the gloves and start again.

7. Holding your gloved hand under the cuff of the glove, insert your other hand into the glove (see figure 13-37D). Keep the thumb of your gloved hand tucked in to avoid possible contamination.
8. Turn the cuffs up by manipulating only the sterile surface of the gloves (sterile touches sterile). Go up under the folded cuffs, pull out slightly, and turn cuffs over and up (see figure 13-37E.) Do not touch the inside of the gloves or the skin with your gloved hand.
9. Interlace the fingers to position the gloves correctly, taking care not to touch the skin with the gloved hands (see figure 13-37F).

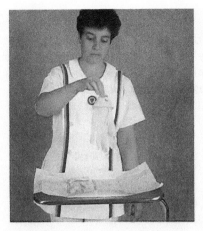

FIGURE 13-37A Pick up the first glove by grasping the glove on the top edge of the folded-down cuff.

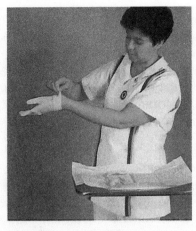

FIGURE 13-37B Hold the glove securely by the cuff and slip the opposite hand into the glove.

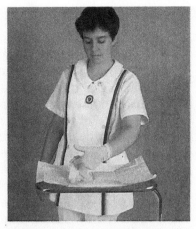

FIGURE 13-37C Slip the gloved fingers under the cuff of the second glove to lift it from the package.

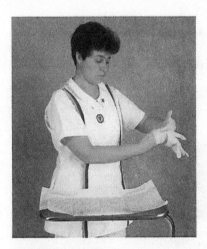

FIGURE 13-37D Hold the gloved hand under the cuff while inserting the other hand into the glove.

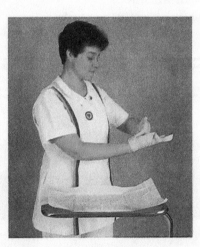

FIGURE 13-37E Insert the gloved fingers under the cuff, pull out slightly, and turn the cuffs over and up without touching the inside of the gloves or the skin.

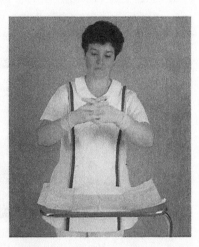

FIGURE 13-37F Interlace the fingers to position the gloves correctly, taking care not to touch the skin with the gloved hands.

CAUTION: If contamination occurs, start again with a new pair of gloves.

10. Do not touch anything that is not sterile once the gloves are in place. Gloves are applied for the purpose of performing procedures requiring sterile technique. During any procedure they become contaminated with organisms related to the patient's condition, for example, wound drainage, blood, or other body discharges. Even a clean, dry wound may contaminate gloves.

NOTE: Gloved hands should remain in position above the waist. Do *not* allow them to fall below waist.

11. After the procedure requiring sterile gloves is completed, dispose of all contaminated supplies before removing gloves.

NOTE: This reduces the danger of cross-infection caused by handling contaminated supplies without glove protection.

12. To remove the gloves, use one gloved hand to grasp the other glove by the outside of the

cuff. Taking care not to touch the skin, remove the glove by pulling it down over the hand. It will be wrong side out when removed.

NOTE: This prevents contamination of your hands by organisms picked up during performance of the procedure. Now you must consider the outside of the gloves contaminated, and the area inside, next to your skin, clean.

13. Insert your bare fingers on the inside of the second glove. Remove the glove by pulling it down gently, taking care not to touch the outside of the glove with your bare fingers. It will be wrong side out when removed.

   ⓘ CAUTION: Avoid touching your uniform or any other object with the contaminated gloves.

14. Put the contaminated gloves in an infectious waste container immediately after removal.

15. Wash your hands immediately and thoroughly after removing gloves.

16. Once the gloves have been removed, do not handle any contaminated equipment or supplies such as soiled dressings or drainage basins. Protect yourself.

17. Replace equipment if necessary.

18. Wash hands thoroughly.

Practice *Go to the workbook and use the evaluation sheet for 13:7C, Donning and Removing Sterile Gloves, to practice this procedure. When you feel you have mastered this skill, sign the sheet and give it to your instructor for further action.*

 Final Checkpoint Using the criteria listed on the evaluation sheet, your instructor will grade your performance.

PROCEDURE 13:7D
Changing a Sterile Dressing

Equipment and Supplies

Sterile tray with basin, solution, gauze sponges and pads (or a prepared sterile dressing package); sterile gloves; adhesive or nonallergic tape; disposable gloves; infectious waste bag

Procedure

1. Check doctor's written orders or obtain orders from immediate supervisor.
   NOTE: Dressings should *not* be changed without orders.
   NOTE: The policy of your agency will determine how you obtain orders for procedures.

2. Assemble equipment. Check autoclave indicator and date on all equipment. If more than 30 days have elapsed, use another package with a more recent date. Put the unsterile package aside for resterilization.

3. Wash hands thoroughly.

4. Prepare a sterile tray as previously taught (in Procedure 13:7B) or obtain a commercially prepared sterile dressing package.
   NOTE: Prepared packages are used in some agencies.
   ⓘ CAUTION: Never let the tray out of your sight once it has been prepared.

5. Take all necessary equipment to the patient area. Place it where it will be convenient for use yet free from possible contamination by other equipment, for example, an uncluttered bedside tray or stand.

6. Introduce yourself. Identify the patient. Explain the procedure. Close the door and/or windows to avoid drafts and flow of organisms into the room.

7. Screen the unit or draw curtains to provide privacy for the patient. If the patient is in a bed, elevate the bed to a comfortable working height and lower the siderail. Expose the body area needing the dressing change. Use

sheets or drapes as necessary to prevent unnecessary exposure of the patient.

8. Fold down a 2- to 3-inch cuff on the top of the infectious waste bag. Position it in a convenient location. Tear off the tape you will need later to secure the clean dressing. Place it in an area where it will be available for easy access.

9. ☣ Put on disposable, nonsterile gloves. Gently but firmly remove the tape from the soiled dressing. Discard it in the infectious waste bag. Hold the skin taut and then lift the dressing carefully, taking care not to pull on any surgical drains. Note the type, color, and amount of drainage on the dressing. Discard dressing in the infectious waste bag.

   NOTE: Surgical drains are placed in some surgical incisions to aid the removal of secretions. Care must be taken to avoid moving the drains when the dressing is removed.

10. Check the incision site. Observe the type and amount of remaining drainage, color of drainage, and degree of healing.

   ⚠ Ⓒ CAUTION: Report any unusual observations immediately to your supervisor. Examples are bright-red blood, pus, swelling, or abnormal discharges at the wound site or patient complaints of pain or dizziness.

11. Remove disposable gloves and place in infectious waste bag. Immediately wash your hands.

   ⚠ CAUTION: Nonsterile disposable gloves should be worn while removing dressings to avoid contamination of the hands or skin by blood or body discharge.

12. Fanfold the towel back to uncover the sterile tray.

   ⚠ CAUTION: Handle only the contaminated (outside) side of the towel. The side in contact with the tray's contents is the sterile side.

   NOTE: If a prepared package is used, open it at this time.

13. Don sterile gloves as previously taught in Procedure 13:7C.

14. Using thumb and forefinger, pick up a gauze sponge from the basin. Squeeze it slightly to remove any excess solution. Warn the patient that the solution may be cool.

15. Cleanse the wound. Use a circular motion (see figure 13-38).

NOTE: Begin near the center of the wound and move outward or away from the wound. Make an ever-widening circle. Discard the wet gauze sponge after use. Never go back over the same area with the same gauze sponge. Repeat this procedure until the area is clean, using a new gauze sponge each time.

16. Do not cleanse directly over the wound unless there is a great deal of drainage or it is specifically ordered by the physician. If this is to be done, use sterile gauze and wipe with a single stroke from the top to the bottom. Discard the soiled gauze. Repeat as necessary, using a new sterile gauze sponge each time.

17. The wound is now ready for clean dressings. Lift the sterile dressings from the tray and place them lightly on the wound. Make sure they are centered over the wound.

   NOTE: The inner dressing is usually made up of 4- by 4-inch gauze sponges.

18. Apply outer dressings until the wound is sufficiently protected.

   NOTE: Heavier dressings such as abdominal pads are usually used.

   NOTE: The number and size of dressings needed to dress the wound will depend on the amount of drainage and the size of the wound.

19. Remove the sterile gloves as previously taught. Discard them in the infectious waste bag. Immediately wash your hands.

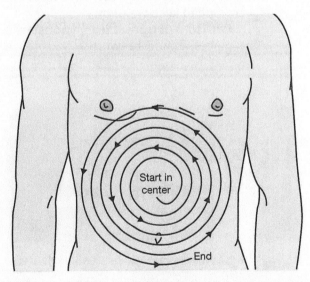

FIGURE 13-38 Use a circular motion to clean the wound, starting at the center of the wound and moving in an outward direction.

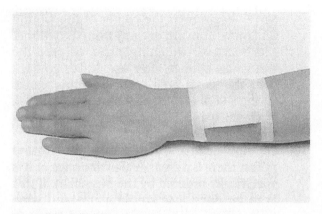

FIGURE 13-39 Tape should be applied so that it runs opposite to body action or movement.

20. Place the precut tape over the dressing at the proper angle. Check to make sure that the dressing is secure and the ends are closed.

    NOTE: Tape should be applied so it runs opposite from body action or movement (see figure 13-39). It should be the correct width for the dressing. It should be long enough to support the dressing, but it should not be too long because it will irritate the patient's skin.

21. Check to be sure the patient is comfortable and that safety precautions have been observed before leaving the area.

22. Put on disposable, nonsterile gloves. Clean and replace all equipment used. Tie or tape the infectious waste bag securely. Dispose of it according to agency policy.

    CAUTION: Disposable, nonsterile gloves should be worn to provide a protective barrier while cleaning equipment or supplies that may be contaminated by blood or body fluids.

23. Remove disposable gloves. Wash hands thoroughly. Protect yourself from possible contamination.

24. C Record the following information on the patient's chart or agency form: date, time, dressing change, amount and type of drainage, and any other pertinent information, or tell this information to your immediate supervisor.

    Example: 1/8/—, 9:00 A.M. Dressing changed on right abdominal area. Small amount of thick, light-yellow discharge noted on dressings. No swelling or inflammation apparent at incision site. Sterile dressing applied. Your signature and title.

    NOTE: Report any unusual observations immediately.

Practice *Go to the workbook and use the evaluation sheet for 13:7D, Changing a Sterile Dressing, to practice this procedure. When you feel you have mastered this skill, sign the sheet and give it to your instructor for further action.*

Final Checkpoint Using the criteria listed on the evaluation sheet, your instructor will grade your performance.

13:8 INFORMATION Maintaining Transmission-Based Isolation Precautions

OBRA In health occupations, you will deal with many different diseases/disorders. Some diseases are communicable and require isolation. A **communicable disease** is caused by a pathogenic organism that can be easily transmitted to others.

 Transmission-based isolation precautions are a method or technique of caring for patients who have communicable diseases. Examples of communicable diseases are tuberculosis, wound infections, and pertussis (whooping cough). Standard precautions, discussed in Information Section 13:3, do not eliminate the need for specific transmission-based isolation precautions. Standard precautions are used on all patients. Transmission-based isolation techniques are used to provide extra protection against specific diseases or pathogens to prevent their spread.

Communicable diseases are spread in many ways. Some examples include direct contact with the patient; contact with dirty linen, equipment, and/or supplies; and contact with blood, body fluids, secretions, and excretions such as urine, feces, droplets (from sneezing, coughing, or spitting), and discharges from wounds. Transmission-based isolation precautions are used to limit contact with pathogenic organisms. These techniques help prevent the spread of the disease to other people and protect patients, their families, and health care providers.

The type of transmission-based isolation used depends on the causative organism of the disease, the way the organism is transmitted, and whether or not the pathogen is antibiotic-resistant (not affected by antibiotics). Personal protective equipment (PPE) is used to provide protection from the pathogen. Some transmission-based isolation precautions require the use of gowns, gloves, face shields, and masks (see figure 13-40), while others only require the use of a mask.

Two terms are extensively used in transmission-based isolation: *contaminated* and *clean*. These words refer to the presence of organisms on objects.

◆ **Contaminated,** or dirty, means that objects contain disease-producing organisms. These objects must not be touched, unless the health worker is protected by gloves, gown, and other required items.
   NOTE: The outside and waist ties of the gown, protective gloves, and mask are considered contaminated.

◆ **Clean** means that objects or parts of objects do *not* contain disease-producing organisms and therefore have minimal chance of spreading the disease. Every effort must be made to prevent contamination of these objects or parts of objects.
   NOTE: The insides of the gloves and gown are clean, as are the neckband, its ties, and the mask ties.

The Centers for Disease Control and Prevention (CDC) in conjunction with the National Center for Infectious Diseases (NCID) and the Hospital Infection Control Practices Advisory Committee (HICPAC) has recommended four

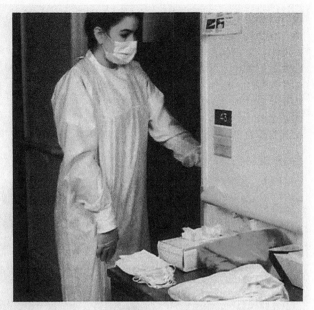

FIGURE 13-40 Some transmission-based isolation precautions require the use of gowns, gloves, and a mask, while others only require the use of a mask.

main classifications of precautions that must be followed: standard, airborne, droplet, and contact. Health care facilities are provided with a list of infections/conditions that shows the type and duration of precautions needed for each specific disease. In this way, facilities can follow the guidelines to determine the type of transmission-based isolation that should be used along with the specific precautions that must be followed.

Standard precautions (discussed in Information Section 13:3), are used on all patients. In addition, a patient must be placed in a private room if the patient contaminates the environment or does not (or cannot be expected to) assist in maintaining appropriate hygiene. Every health care worker must be well informed about standard precautions and follow the recommendations for the use of gloves, gowns, and face masks when conditions indicate their use.

Airborne precautions (see figure 13-41), are used for patients known or suspected to be infected with pathogens transmitted by airborne droplet nuclei, small particles of evaporated droplets that contain microorganisms and remain suspended in the air or on dust particles. Examples of diseases requiring these isolation precautions are rubella (measles), varicella (chicken pox), tuberculosis, and shingles or herpes zoster (varicella-zoster). In addition to using standard precautions, several other precautions are required. The patient must be placed in a private room, and the door should be kept closed. Air in the room must be discharged to outdoor air or filtered before being circulated to other areas. Each person who enters the room must wear respiratory protection in the form of a N95, P100 or more powerful filtering mask such as a high-efficiency particulate air (HEPA) mask (see figure 13-42A, B). These masks contain special filters to prevent the entrance of the small airborne pathogens. The masks must be fit tested to make sure they create a tight seal each time they are worn by a health care provider. Men with facial hair cannot wear a standard filtering mask because a beard prevents an airtight

AIRBORNE PRECAUTIONS
In Addition to Standard Precautions

Visitors - Report to Nurses' Station Before Entering Room

BEFORE CARE	DURING CARE	AFTER CARE

BEFORE CARE

1. Private room and closed door with monitored negative air pressure, frequent air exchanges, and high-efficiency filtration.

2. Wash hands.

3. Wear respiratory protection appropriate for disease.

DURING CARE

1. Limit transport of patient/resident to essential purposes only. Patient resident must wear mask appropriate for disease.

2. Limit use of noncritical care equipment to a single patient/resident.

AFTER CARE

1. Bag linen to prevent contamination of self, environment, or outside of bag.

2. Discard infectious trash to prevent contamination of self, environment, or outside of bag.

3. Wash hands.

FIGURE 13-41 Airborne precautions. *(Courtesy of Brevis Corporation)*

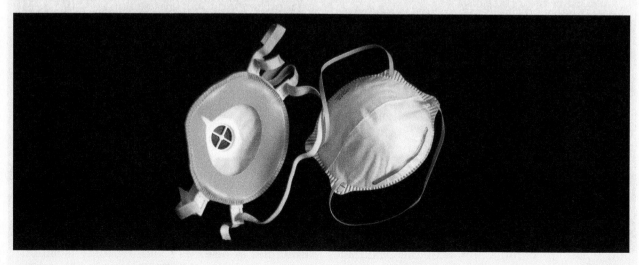

FIGURE 13-42A, B Respirator masks.

seal. Men with facial hair can use a special HEPA-filtered hood. People susceptible to measles or chicken pox should not enter the room. If at all possible, the patient should not be moved from the room. If transport is essential, however, the patient must wear a surgical mask during transport to minimize the release of droplets into the air.

Droplet precautions (see figure 13-43), must be followed for a patient known or suspected to be infected with pathogens transmitted by large-particle droplets expelled during coughing, sneezing, talking, or laughing. Examples of diseases requiring these isolation precautions include *Haemophilus influenzae* meningitis and pneumonia; *Neisseria* meningitis and pneumonia; multidrug-resistant *Streptococcus* meningitis, pneumonia, sinusitis, and otitis media; diphtheria; *Mycoplasma* pneumonia; pertussis; adenovirus; mumps; and severe viral influenza. In addition to using standard precautions, the patient should be placed in a private room. If a private room is not available and the patient cannot be placed in a room with a patient who has the same infection, a distance of at least 3 feet should separate the infected patient and other patients or visitors. Masks

must be worn when working within three feet of the patient, and the use of masks anywhere in the room is strongly recommended. If transport or movement of the patient is essential, the patient must wear a surgical mask.

Contact precautions (see figure 13-44), must be followed for any patients known or suspected to be infected with *epidemiologically* (capable of spreading rapidly from person to person, an epidemic) important microorganisms that can be transmitted by either direct or indirect contact. Examples of diseases requiring these precautions include any gastrointestinal, respiratory, skin, or wound infections caused by multidrug-resistant organisms; diapered or incontinent patients with enterohemorrhagic *E. coli*, *Shigella*, hepatitis A, or rotavirus; viral or hemorrhagic conjunctivitis or fevers; and any skin infections that are highly contagious or that may occur on dry skin, such as diphtheria, herpes simplex virus, impetigo, pediculosis (head or body lice), scabies, and staphylococcal infections. In addition to using standard precautions, the patient should be placed in a private room or, if a private room is not available, in a room with a patient who has an active infection caused by the same organism. Gloves must be

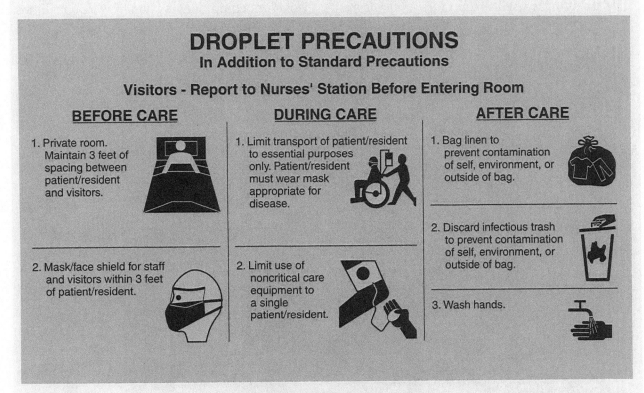

FIGURE 13-43 Droplet precautions. *(Courtesy of Brevis Corporation)*

worn when entering the room. Gloves must be changed after having contact with any material that may contain high concentrations of the microorganism, such as wound drainage or fecal material. Gloves must be removed before leaving the room, and the hands must be washed with an antimicrobial agent. A gown must be worn in the room if there is any chance of contact with the patient, environmental surfaces, or items in the room. The gown must be removed before leaving the room and care must be taken to ensure that clothing is not contaminated after gown removal. Movement and transport of the patient from the room should be for essential purposes only. The room and items in it must receive daily cleaning and disinfection as needed. If possible, patient-care equipment (bedside commode, stethoscope, sphygmomanometer, thermometer) should be left in the room and used only for this patient. If this is not possible, all equipment must be cleaned and disinfected before being used on another patient.

Protective or **reverse isolation** refers to methods used to protect certain patients from organisms present in the environment. Protective isolation is used mainly for *immunocom-promised* patients, or those whose body defenses are not capable of protecting them from infections and disease. Examples of patients requiring this protection are patients whose immune systems have been depressed prior to receiving transplants (such as bone marrow transplants), severely burned patients, patients receiving chemotherapy or radiation treatments, or patients whose immune systems have failed. Precautions vary depending on the patient's condition. The patient is usually placed in a room that has been cleaned and disinfected. Frequent disinfection occurs while the patient occupies the room. Many facilities require anyone entering the room to wear clean or sterile gowns, gloves, and masks. All equipment or supplies brought into the room are clean, disinfected, and/or sterile. Special filters may be used to purify air that enters the room. Every effort is made to protect the patient from microorganisms that cause infection or disease.

Exact procedures for maintaining transmission-based isolation precautions vary from one facility to another. The procedures used depend on the type of units provided for isolation patients, and on the kind of supplies or special isolation equipment available. Most facilities

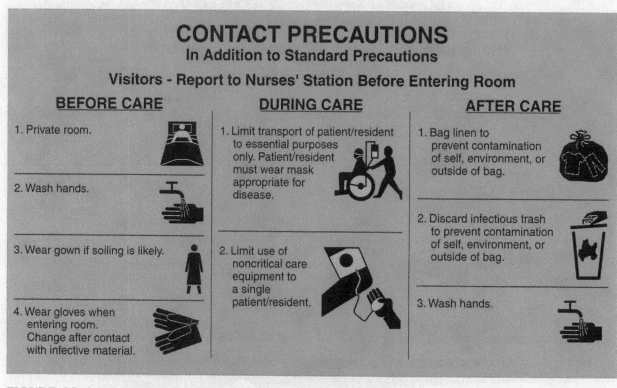

FIGURE 13-44 Contact precautions. *(Courtesy of Brevis Corporation)*

convert a regular patient room into an isolation room, but some facilities use special, two-room isolation units. Some facilities use disposable supplies such as gloves, gowns, and treatment packages. Therefore, it is essential that you learn the isolation procedure followed by your agency. However, the basic principles for maintaining transmission-based isolation are the same regardless of the facility. Therefore, if you know these basic principles, you will be able to adjust to any setting.

STUDENT: *Go to the workbook and complete the assignment sheet for 13:8, Maintaining Transmission-Based Isolation Precautions. Then return and continue with the procedures.*

PROCEDURE 13:8A

Donning and Removing Transmission-Based Isolation Garments

OBRA **NOTE:** The following procedure deals with contact transmission-based isolation precautions. For other types of transmission-based isolation, follow only the steps that apply.

Equipment and Supplies

Isolation gown, surgical mask, gloves, small plastic bag, linen cart or container, infectious waste container, paper towels, sink with running water

Procedure

1. Assemble equipment.
   NOTE: In many agencies, clean isolation garments and supplies are kept available on a cart outside the isolation unit, or in the outer room of a two-room unit. A waste container should be positioned just inside the door.
2. Wash hands.
3. Remove rings and place them in your pocket or pin them to your uniform.
4. Remove your watch and place it in a small plastic bag or centered on a clean paper towel. If placed on a towel, handle only the bottom part of the towel; do not touch the top.
   NOTE: The watch will be taken into the room and placed on the bedside stand for taking vital signs. Because it cannot be sterilized, it must be kept clean.
   NOTE: In some agencies, a plastic-covered watch is left in the isolation room.

5. Put on the mask. Secure it under your chin. Make sure to cover your mouth and nose. Handle the mask as little as possible. Tie the mask securely behind your head and neck. Tie the top ties first and the bottom ties second.
   NOTE: The tie bands on the mask are considered clean. The mask is considered contaminated.
   NOTE: The mask is considered to be contaminated after 30 minutes in isolation or anytime it gets wet. If you remain in isolation longer than 30 minutes, or if the mask gets wet, you must wash your hands, and remove and discard the old mask. Then wash your hands again, and put on a clean mask.
6. If uniform sleeves are long, roll them up above the elbows before putting on the gown.
7. Lift the gown by placing your hands inside the shoulders (see figure 13-45A).
   NOTE: The inside of the gown and the ties at the neck are considered clean.
   NOTE: Most agencies use disposable gowns that are discarded after use.
8. Work your arms into the sleeves of the gown by gentle twisting. Take care not to touch your face with the sleeves of the gown.
9. Place your hands *inside* the neckband, adjust until it is in position, and then tie the bands at the back of your neck (see figure 13-45B).
10. Reach behind and fold the edges of the gown over so that the uniform is completely

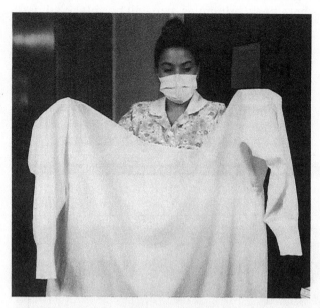

FIGURE 13-45A After tying the mask in place, put on the gown by placing your hands inside the shoulders.

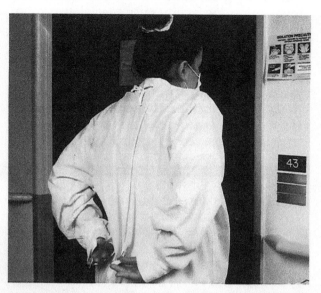

FIGURE 13-45C Overlap the back edges of the gown so your uniform is completely covered before tying the waist ties.

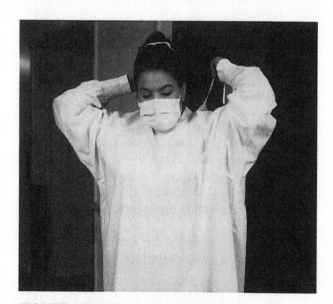

FIGURE 13-45B Slip your fingers inside the neckband to tie the gown at the neck.

covered. Tie the waistbands (see figure 13-45C). Some waistbands are long enough to wrap around your body before tying.

11. If gloves are to be worn, put them on. Make sure that the cuff of the glove comes over the top of the cuff of the gown. In this way, there are no open areas for entrance of organisms.

12. You are now ready to enter the isolation room. Double check to be sure you have all equipment and supplies that you will need for patient care before you enter the room.

13. When patient care is complete, you will be ready to remove isolation garments. In a two-room isolation unit, go to the outer room. In a one-room unit, remove garments while you are standing close to the inside of the door. Take care to avoid touching the room's contaminated articles.

14. Untie the waist ties. Loosen the gown at the waist.
    NOTE: The waist ties are considered contaminated.

15. If gloves are worn, remove the first glove by grasping the outside of the cuff with the opposite gloved hand. Pull the glove over the hand so that the glove is inside out. Remove the second glove by placing the bare hand inside the cuff. Pull the glove off so it is inside out. Place the disposable gloves in the infectious waste container.

16. To avoid unnecessary transmission of organisms, use paper towels to turn on the water faucet. Wash and dry your hands thoroughly. When they are dry, use a clean, dry paper towel to turn off the faucet.
    ⚠ CAUTION: Organisms travel rapidly through wet towels.

17. Untie the mask. Holding the mask by the ties only, drop it into the infectious waste container.

NOTE: The ties of the mask are considered clean. Do not touch any other part of the mask because it is considered contaminated.

18. Untie the neck ties. Loosen the gown at the shoulders, handling only the inside of the gown.

NOTE: The neck ties are considered clean.

19. Slip the fingers of one hand inside the opposite cuff. Do *not* touch the outside. Pull the sleeve down over the hand (see figure 13-46A).

⚠ CAUTION: The outside of the gown is considered contaminated and should not be touched.

20. Using the gown-covered hand, pull the sleeve down over the opposite hand (see figure 13-46B).

21. Ease your arms and hands out of the gown. Keep the gown in front of your body and keep your hands away from the outside of the gown. Use as gentle a motion as possible.

NOTE: Excessive flapping of the gown will spread organisms.

22. With your hands inside the gown at the shoulders, bring the shoulders together and turn the gown so that it is inside out (see figure 13-46C). In this manner, the outside of the contaminated gown is on the inside. Fold the gown in half and then roll it together. Place it in the infectious waste container.

NOTE: Avoid excess motion during this procedure because motion causes the spread of organisms.

23. Wash hands thoroughly. Use dry, clean paper towels to operate the faucets.

24. Touch only the inside of the plastic bag to remove your watch. Discard the bag in the waste container. If the watch is on a paper towel, handle only the "clean," top portion (if necessary). Discard the towel in the infectious waste container.

25. Use a clean paper towel to open the door. Discard the towel in the waste container before leaving the room.

⚠ CAUTION: The inside of the door is considered contaminated.

NOTE: The waste container should be positioned just inside the door of the room.

26. After leaving the isolation room, wash hands thoroughly. This will help prevent spread of the disease. It also protects you from the illness.

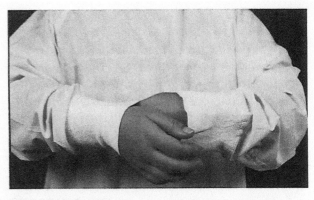

FIGURE 13-46A To remove the gown, slip the fingers of one hand under the cuff of the opposite arm to pull the gown down over the opposite hand.

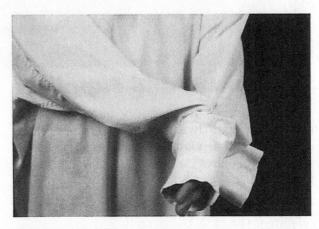

FIGURE 13-46B Using the gown-covered hand, grasp the outside of the gown on the opposite arm and pull the gown down over the hand.

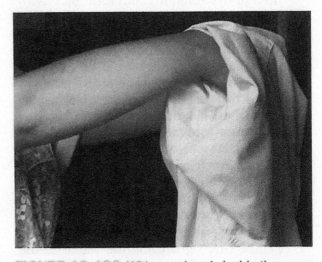

FIGURE 13-46C With your hands inside the gown at the shoulders, bring the shoulders together and turn the gown so that it is inside out, with the contaminated side on the inside.

Practice *Go to the workbook and use the evaluation sheet for 13:8A, Donning and Removing Transmission-Based Isolation Garments, to practice this procedure. When you feel you have mastered this skill, sign the sheet and give it to your instructor for further action.*

 Final Checkpoint Using the criteria listed on the evaluation sheet, your instructor will grade your performance.

PROCEDURE 13:8B

Working in a Hospital Transmission-Based Isolation Unit

Equipment and Supplies

Clothes hamper, two laundry bags, two trays, dishes, cups, bowls, waste container lined with a plastic bag, infectious waste bags, bags, tape, pencil, pen, paper

Procedure

1. Assemble all equipment.
    NOTE: Any equipment or supplies to be used in the isolation room must be assembled prior to entering the room.
2. Wash hands.
3. Put on appropriate isolation garments as previously instructed.
4. Tape paper to the outside of the isolation door. This will be used to record vital signs.
5. Enter the isolation room. Take all needed equipment into the room.
6. Introduce yourself. Greet and identify patient. Provide patient care as needed.
    NOTE: All care is provided in a routine manner. However, transmission-based isolation garments must be worn as ordered.
7. To record vital signs:
    a. Take vital signs using the watch in the plastic bag. (If the watch is not in a plastic bag, hold it with the bottom part of a paper towel.) Use other equipment in the room as needed.
    b. Open the door touching only the inside, or contaminated side.
    c. Using a pencil, record the vital signs on the paper taped to the door. Do *not* touch the outside of the door at any time.
    NOTE: The pencil remains in the room because it is contaminated.
8. To transfer food into the isolation unit:
    a. Transfer of food requires two people; one person must stay outside the unit and one inside.
    b. The person inside the isolation unit picks up the empty tray in the room and opens door, touching only the inside of the door.
    c. The person outside hands in the cups, bowls, and plates of food.
    d. When transferring food, the two people should handle the opposite sides of the dishes. In this manner, one person will not touch the other person.
    e. Glasses should be held near the top by the transfer person on the outside. The transfer person on the inside should receive the glasses by holding them on the bottom.
9. To dispose of leftover food or waste:
    a. Liquids can be poured down the sink or flushed down the toilet.
    b. Soft foods such as mashed potatoes or cooked vegetables can be flushed down the toilet.
    c. Hard particles of food, such as bone, should be placed in the plastic-lined trash container.
    d. Disposable utensils or dishes should be placed in the plastic-lined trash container.

e. Metal utensils should be washed and kept in the isolation room to be used as needed for other meals. These utensils, however, are contaminated. When they are removed from the isolation room, they must be disinfected or double bagged and labeled before being sent for decontamination and reprocessing.

10. To transfer soiled linen from the unit, two people are required:
a. All dirty linen should be folded and rolled.
b. Place linen in the linen hamper.
c. Person outside the unit should cuff the top of a clean infectious waste laundry bag and hold it. Hands should be kept on the inside of the bag's cuff to avoid contamination.
d. Person in isolation should seal the isolation bag. The bag is then placed inside the outer bag, which is being held by the person outside.
e. Outer bag should be folded over at the top and taped by the person outside. The bag should be labeled as "BIOHAZARDOUS LINEN."
f. At all times, no direct contact should occur between the two people transferring linen. NOTE: Many agencies use special isolation linen bags. Hot water dissolves the bags during the washing process. Therefore, no other personnel handle the contaminated linen after it leaves the isolation unit.

11. To transfer trash from the isolation unit, two people are required:
a. Any trash in the isolation room should be in plastic bags. Any trash or disposable items contaminated with blood, body fluids, secretions, or excretions should be placed in infectious waste bags.
b. When the bag is full, expel excess air by pushing gently on the bag.
c. Tie a knot at the top of the bag to seal it or fold the top edge twice and tape it securely.
d. Place this bag inside a cuffed biohazardous waste bag held by a "clean" person outside the unit.
e. The outside person then ties the outer bag securely or tapes the outer bag shut.
f. The double-bagged trash should then be burned. Double-bagged infectious waste is autoclaved prior to incineration or disposal as infectious waste according to legal requirements.

g. At all times, direct contact between the two people transferring trash must be avoided.

12. To transfer equipment from the isolation unit two people are required:
a. Thoroughly clean and disinfect all equipment in the unit.
b. After cleaning, place equipment in a plastic bag or special isolation bag. Label the bag with the contents and the word "ISOLATION."
c. After folding the bag down twice at the top, tape the bag shut.
d. A second person outside the isolation room should hold a second, cuffed infectious waste bag.
e. The person in isolation places the sealed, contaminated bag inside the bag being held outside the unit. The person in isolation should have no direct contact with the clean bag.
f. The person outside the unit turns down the top of the infectious waste bag twice and securely tapes the bag. The outside person then labels the bag with the contents, for example, "ISOLATION DISHES."
g. The double-bagged material is then sent to Central Supply or another designated area for sterilization and/or decontamination.

13. The transmission-based isolation unit must be kept clean and neat at all times. Equipment no longer needed should be transferred out of the unit using the appropriate isolation technique.

14. Before leaving an isolation room, ask the patient whether a urinal or bedpan is needed. This will save time and energy by reducing the need to return to provide additional patient care shortly after leaving. Also, prior to leaving, check all safety and comfort points to make sure patient care is complete.

15. Remove isolation garments as previously instructed (in Procedure 13:8A).

16. Wash hands thoroughly.

Practice *Go to the workbook and use the evaluation sheet for 13:8B, Working in a Hospital Transmission-Based Isolation Unit, to practice this procedure. When you feel you have mastered this skill, sign the sheet and give it to your instructor for further action.*

CHAPTER 3
Vital Signs

Introduction

After completing this unit of study, you should be able to:

◆ List the four main vital signs
◆ Convert Fahrenheit temperatures to Celsius, or Celsius to Fahrenheit
◆ Read a clinical thermometer to the nearest two-tenths of a degree
◆ Measure and record oral temperature accurately
◆ Measure and record rectal temperature accurately
◆ Measure and record axillary temperature accurately
◆ Measure and record tympanic (aural) temperature accurately
◆ Measure and record radial pulse to an accuracy within ± 2 beats per minute
◆ Count and record respirations to an accuracy within ± 1 respiration per minute
◆ Measure and record apical pulse to an accuracy within ± 2 beats per minute
◆ Measure and record blood pressure to an accuracy within ± 2 mm of actual mercury reading
◆ State the normal range for oral temperature, axillary temperature, rectal temperature, pulse, respirations, systolic pressure, and diastolic pressure
◆ Define, pronounce, and spell all the key terms

 Observe Standard Precautions

 Safety—Proceed with Caution

 Math Skill

 Science Skill

C Communications Skill

 Instructors Check—Call Instructor at This Point

 OBRA OBRA Requirement—Based on Federal Law

 Legal Responsibility

 Career Information

 Technology

KEY TERMS

apical pulse
   (ape'-ih-kal)

apnea
   (ap'-nee"-ah)

arrhythmia
   (ah-rith'-me-ah)

aural

axillary

blood pressure

bradycardia
   (bray"-dee-car'-dee-ah)

bradypnea
   (brad"-ip-nee'-ah)

character

Cheyne–Stokes
   (chain' stokes")

clinical thermometers

cyanosis

diastolic
   (die"-ah-stall'-ik)

dyspnea
   (dis(p)'-nee"-ah)

electronic thermometers

fever

homeostasis
   (home"-ee-oh-stay'-sis)

hypertension

hyperthermia
   (high-pur-therm'-ee-ah)

hypotension

hypothermia
   (high-po-therm'-ee-ah)

oral

orthopnea
   (or"-thop-nee'-ah)

pulse

pulse deficit

pulse pressure

pyrexia

rale *(rawl)*

rate

rectal

respirations

rhythm

sphygmomanometer
   (sfig"-moh-ma-nam'-eh-ter)

stethoscope
   (steth'-uh-scope)

systolic
   (sis"-tall'-ik)

tachycardia
   (tack"-eh-car'-dee-ah)

tachypnea
   (tack"-ip-nee'-ah)

temperature

tympanic thermometers

vital signs

volume

wheezing

14:1 INFORMATION Measuring and Recording Vital Signs

Vital signs are important indicators of health states of the body. This unit discusses all of the vital signs in detail. The basic information that follows serves as an introduction for this topic.

Vital signs are defined as various determinations that provide information about the basic body conditions of the patient. The four main vital signs are temperature, pulse, respirations, and blood pressure. Many health care professionals are now regarding the degree of pain as the fifth vital sign. Patients are asked to rate their level of pain on a scale of 1 to 10, with 1 being minimal pain and 10 being severe pain. Other important vital signs that provide information about the patient's condition include the color of the skin, the size of the pupils in the eyes and their reaction to light, the level of consciousness, and the patient's response to stimuli. As a health care worker, it will be your responsibility to measure and record the vital signs of patients. However, it is not in your realm of duties to reveal this information to the patient. The physician will decide if the patient should be given this information. It is essential that vital signs be accurate. They are often the first indication of a disease or abnormality in the patient.

Temperature is a measurement of the balance between heat lost and heat produced by the body. Temperature can be

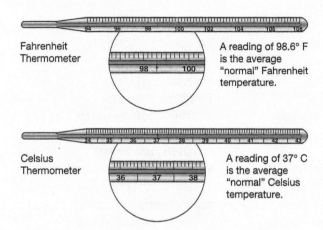

FIGURE 14-1 Normal oral body temperature on Fahrenheit and Celsius thermometers.

measured in the mouth (oral), rectum (rectal), armpit (axillary), or ear (aural). A low or high reading can indicate disease. Most temperatures are measured in degrees on a thermometer that has a Fahrenheit scale. However, some health care facilities are now measuring temperature in degrees on a Celsius (centigrade) scale. A comparison of the two scales is shown in figure 14-1 and in Appendix B. At times, it may be necessary to convert Fahrenheit temperatures to Celsius, or Celsius to Fahrenheit. The formulas for the conversion are as follows:

◆ To convert Fahrenheit (F) temperatures to Celsius (C) temperatures, subtract 32 from the Fahrenheit temperature and then multiply the result by 5/9, or 0.5556. For example, to convert a Fahrenheit temperature of 212 to Celsius, subtract 32 from 212 to get 180. Then multiply 180 by 5/9, or 0.5556, to get the Celsius temperature of 100.0.

◆ To convert Celsius (C) temperatures to Fahrenheit (F) temperatures, multiply the Celsius temperature by 9/5, or 1.8, and then add 32 to the total. For example, to convert a Celsius temperature of 37 to Fahrenheit, multiply 37 by 9/5, or 1.8, to get 66.6. Then add 32 to 66.6 to get the Fahrenheit temperature of 98.6.

Pulse is the pressure of the blood felt against the wall of an artery as the heart contracts and relaxes, or beats. The rate, rhythm, and volume are recorded. **Rate** refers to the number of beats per minute, **rhythm** refers to regularity, and **volume** refers to strength. The pulse is usually taken over the radial artery, although it may be felt over any superficial artery that has a bone behind it. Any abnormality can indicate disease.

Respirations reflect the breathing rate of the patient. In addition to the respiration count, the rhythm (regularity) and character (type) of respirations are noted. Abnormal respirations usually indicate that a health problem or disease is present.

Blood pressure is the force exerted by the blood against the arterial walls when the heart contracts or relaxes. Two readings (systolic and diastolic) are noted to show the greatest pressure and the least pressure. Both are very important. Abnormal blood pressure is often the first indication of disease.

Another vital sign is the **apical pulse.** This pulse is taken with a stethoscope at the apex of the heart. The actual heartbeat is heard and counted. At times, because of illness, hardening of the arteries, a weak or very rapid radial pulse, or doctor's orders, you will be required to take an apical pulse. Also, because infants and small children have a very rapid radial pulse that is difficult to count, apical pulses are usually taken.

C If you note any abnormality or change in any vital sign, it is your responsibility to report this immediately to your supervisor. If you have difficulty obtaining a correct reading, ask another individual to check the patient. Never guess, or report an inaccurate reading.

STUDENT: *Go to the workbook and complete the assignment sheet for 14:1, Measuring and Recording Vital Signs.*

14:2 INFORMATION Measuring and Recording Temperature

OBRA Body temperature is one of the main vital signs. This section provides the basic guidelines for taking and recording temperature.

Temperature is defined as "the balance between heat lost and heat produced by the body." Heat is lost through perspiration, respiration, and excretion (urine and feces). Heat is produced by the metabolism of food, and by muscle and gland activity. A constant state of fluid balance, known as **homeostasis**, is the ideal health state in the human body. The rates of chemical reactions in the body are regulated by body temperature. Therefore, if body temperature is too high or too low, the body's fluid balance is affected.

The normal range for body temperature is 97° to 100° Fahrenheit, or 36.1° to 37.8° Celsius (sometimes called centigrade). However, variations in body temperature can occur, as noted in the following information:

◆ Individuals have different body temperatures. Some people have accelerated body processes and, thus, usually have higher temperatures. Others have slower body processes and, thus, lower temperatures.

◆ Time of day also affects body temperature. Body temperature is usually lower in the morning, after the body has rested. It is higher in the evening, after muscular activity and daily food intake have taken place.

◆ Parts of the body where temperatures are taken lead to variations. Temperature variations by body site are shown in table 14-1.

(1) **Oral** temperatures are taken in the mouth. The clinical thermometer is left in place for 3 to 5 minutes. This is usually the most common, convenient, and comfortable method of obtaining a temperature.

(2) **Rectal** temperatures are taken in the rectum. The clinical thermometer is left in place for 3 to 5 minutes. This is an internal measurement and is the most accurate of all methods.

(3) An **axillary** temperature is taken in the armpit, under the upper arm. The arm is held close to the body, and the thermometer is inserted between the two folds of skin. A *groin* temperature is taken between the two folds of skin formed by the inner part of the thigh and the lower abdomen. Both axillary and groin are external temperatures and, thus, less accurate. The clinical thermometer is held in place for 10 minutes.

(4) An **aural** temperature is taken with a special thermometer that is placed in the ear or auditory canal. The thermometer detects and measures the thermal, infrared energy radiating from blood vessels in the tympanic membrane, or eardrum. Because this provides a measurement of body core temperature, there is no normal range. Instead, the temperature is calculated by the thermometer into an equivalent of one of four usual settings: equal mode, oral equivalent, rectal equivalent, or core equivalent. The equal mode provides no offset (adjustment) and is recommended for newborns, for whom axillary temperature is often taken. The oral equivalent is calculated with an offset; this mode is used for adults and children over 3 years of age, for whom oral readings are commonly used. The rectal mode is calculated with an offset and is used mainly for infants up to 3 years of age, for whom rectal temperatures are commonly taken. When the rectal mode is used on adults, the temperature

TABLE 14-1 Temperature Variations by Body Site

	ORAL	RECTAL	AXILLARY OR GROIN
Average Temperature	98.6°F (37°C)	99.6°F (37.6°C)	97.6°F (36.4°C)
Normal Range of Temperature	97.6–99.6°F (36.5–37.5°C)	98.6–100.6°F (37–38.1°C)	96.6–98.6°F (36–37°C)

may read higher than average. The core equivalent is calculated with an offset and measures core body temperatures such as those found in the bladder or pulmonary artery. The core equivalent mode should only be used where adult "core" temperatures are commonly used and should not be used for routine vital sign measurements. Most aural thermometers record temperature in less than 2 seconds; so this is a fast and convenient method for obtaining temperature.

♦ Factors that lead to increased body temperature include illness, infection, exercise, excitement, and high temperatures in the environment.

♦ Factors that lead to decreased body temperature include starvation or fasting, sleep, decreased muscle activity, mouth breathing, exposure to cold temperatures in the environment, and certain diseases.

Very low or very high body temperatures are indicative of abnormal conditions. **Hypothermia** is a low body temperature, below 95°F (35°C) measured rectally. It can be caused by prolonged exposure to cold. Death usually occurs if body temperature drops below 93°F (33.9°C) for a period of time. A **fever** is an elevated body temperature, usually above 101°F (38.3°C) measured rectally. **Pyrexia** is another term for fever. The term *febrile* means a fever is present; *afebrile* means no fever is present or the temperature is within the normal range. Fevers are usually caused by infection or injury. **Hyperthermia** occurs when the body temperature exceeds 104°F (40°C) measured rectally. It can be caused by prolonged exposure to hot temperatures, brain damage, and serious infections. Immediate actions must be taken to lower body temperature, because temperatures above 106°F (41.1°C) can quickly lead to convulsions, brain damage, and death.

Clinical thermometers may be used to record temperatures. A clinical thermometer consists of a slender glass tube containing mercury or alcohol with red dye, which expands when exposed to heat. There are different types of clinical thermometers (see figure 14-2). The glass oral thermometer has a long, slender bulb or a blue tip. A security oral thermometer has a shorter, rounder bulb and is usually marked with a blue tip. A rectal thermometer has a short,

stubby, rounded bulb and may be marked with a red tip. In addition, some clinical thermometers have the word "oral" or "rectal" written on their stems. Disposable plastic sheaths may be used to cover the thermometer when it is used on a patient.

If a clinical thermometer containing mercury breaks, the mercury can evaporate and create a toxic vapor that can harm both humans and the environment. Mercury poisoning attacks the central nervous system in humans. Children, especially those under the age of six, are very susceptible. Mercury can contaminate water supplies and build up in the tissues of fish and animals. Therefore, proper cleanup of a broken clinical thermometer is essential. *Never* use a vacuum cleaner or broom to clean up mercury because this will break up the beads of mercury and allow them to vaporize more quickly. *Never* pour mercury down a drain or discard it in a toilet because this causes contamination of the water supply. If a clinical thermometer breaks, close doors to other indoor areas and open the windows in the room with the mercury spill to vent any vapors outside. Put on gloves and use two cards or stiff paper to push the droplets of mercury and broken glass into a plastic container with a tight-fitting lid. If necessary, use an eyedropper to pick up the balls of mercury. Shine a flashlight in the area of the spill because the light will reflect off the shiny mercury beads and make them easier to see. Wipe the entire area with a damp sponge. Then place all cleanup material, including the paper, eyedropper, gloves, and sponge, in the plastic container and label it "Mercury for Recycling." Seal the lid tightly and take the container to a mercury recycling center. Most waste disposal companies will accept mercury for recycling. To discard unbroken mercury thermometers, place the intact thermometer in a

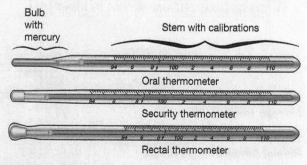

Bulb with mercury

Stem with calibrations

Oral thermometer

Security thermometer

Rectal thermometer

FIGURE 14-2 Types of clinical thermometers.

plastic container with a tight-fitting lid, label it, and take it to a mercury recycling center. To avoid the chance of mercury contamination, the Occupational Health and Safety Administration (OSHA), the Environment Protection Agency (EPA), and the American Medical Association (AMA) recommend the use of alcohol-filled thermometers or digital thermometers.

Electronic thermometers are also used in many facilities. This type of thermometer registers the temperature on a viewer in a few seconds (see figure 14-3). Electronic thermometers can be used to take oral, rectal, axillary, and/or groin temperatures. Most facilities have electronic thermometers with blue probes for oral use and red probes for axillary or rectal use. To prevent cross-contamination, a disposable cover is placed over the thermometer probe

before the temperature is taken. By changing the disposable cover after each use, one unit can be used on many patients. Electronic digital thermometers are excellent for home use because they eliminate the hazard of a mercury spill that occurs when a clinical thermometer is broken (see figure 14-4). The small battery-operated unit usually will register the temperature in about 60 seconds on a digital display screen. Disposable probe covers prevent contamination of the probe. **Tympanic thermometers** are specialized electronic thermometers that record the aural temperature in the ear (see figure 14-5). A disposable plastic cover is placed on the ear probe. By inserting the probe into the auditory canal and pushing a scan button, the temperature is recorded on the screen within 1 to 2 seconds. It is important to read and follow instructions while using this thermometer to obtain an accurate reading.

Plastic or paper thermometers are used in some health care facilities (see figure 14-6). These thermometers contain special chemical dots or strips that change color when exposed to specific temperatures. Some types are placed on the forehead and skin temperature is recorded. Other types are used orally. Both types are used once and discarded.

Electronic and tympanic thermometers are easy to read because they have digital displays. Reading a glass clinical thermometer is a procedure that must be practiced. Hold it at eye level and rotate it slowly to find the solid column of mercury or alcohol (see figure 14-7). Read the thermometer at the point where the mercury or alcohol line ends. Each long line on a

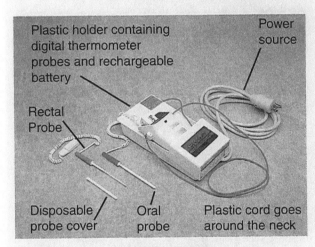

FIGURE 14-3 An electronic thermometer registers the temperature in easy-to-read numbers on a viewer.

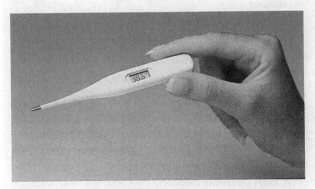

FIGURE 14-4 Electronic digital thermometers are excellent for home use. *(Courtesy of Omron Healthcare Inc., Vernon Hills, IL)*

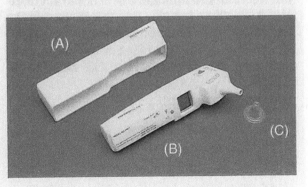

FIGURE 14-5 Tympanic thermometers record the aural temperature in the ear. *Parts include: (A) holder, (B) thermometer, and (C) disposable cover.*

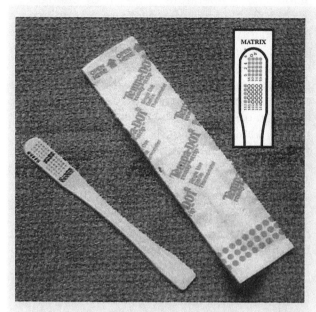

FIGURE 14-6 Plastic disposable thermometers have chemical dots that change color to register body temperature. The matrix shown reads 101°F.

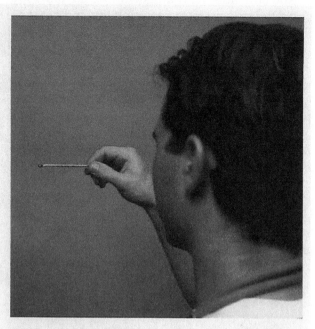

FIGURE 14-7 Hold a clinical thermometer at eye level to find the solid column of mercury or alcohol.

thermometer is read as one degree. An exception to this is the long line for 98.6°F (37°C), which is the normal oral body temperature. Each short line represents 0.2 (two-tenths) of a degree. Temperature is always recorded to the next nearest two-tenths of a degree. In figure 14-8, the line ends at 98.6°F. Top figures explain the markings for each line.

C To record the temperature, write 98^6 instead of 98.6. This reduces the possibility of making an error in reading. For example, a temperature of 100.2 could easily be read as 102. By writing 100^2, the chance of error decreases. If a temperature is taken orally, it is not necessary to indicate that it is an oral reading. If it is taken rectally, place an (R) beside the recording. If it is taken in the axillary area, place an (Ax) beside the recording. If it is taken tympanically (aurally), place a (T) beside the recording. For example:

- 98^6 is an oral reading
- 99^6 (R) is a rectal reading
- 97^6 (Ax) is an axillary reading
- 98^6 (T) is an aural reading

Eating, drinking hot or cold liquids, and/or smoking can alter the temperature in the mouth. It is important to make sure the patient has *not* had anything to eat or drink, or has *not*

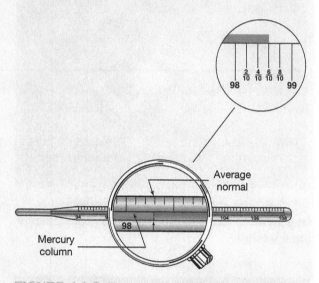

FIGURE 14-8 Each line on a thermometer equals two-tenths of a degree, so the thermometer shown reads 98.6°F.

smoked for at least 15 minutes prior to taking the patient's oral temperature. If the patient has done any of these things, explain why you cannot take the temperature and that you will return to do so.

Thermometers must be cleaned thoroughly after use. The procedure used varies with different agencies. In some agencies, the glass thermometer is washed and rinsed. Cool water is used to prevent breakage and to avoid destroying the column of mercury. The thermometer is then soaked in a disinfectant solution (frequently 70-percent alcohol) for a minimum of 30 minutes before it is used again. Other agencies cover the glass thermometer with a plastic sheath that is discarded after use (see figure 14-9). The probe on electronic thermometers is covered with a plastic sheath that is discarded after each use. These covers prevent the thermometers from coming into contact with each patient's mouth or skin and prevent transmission of germs. Follow your agency's policy for cleaning and care of thermometers.

STUDENT: *Go to the workbook and complete the assignment sheet for 14:2, Measuring and Recording Temperature. Then return and continue with the procedures.*

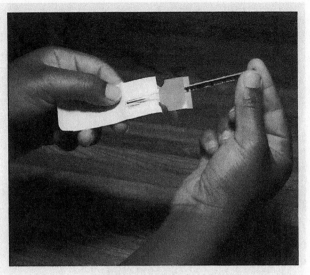

FIGURE 14-9 A clinical thermometer can be covered with a plastic sheath that is discarded after each use.

PROCEDURE 14:2A   OBRA

Cleaning a Clinical Thermometer

Equipment and Supplies

Thermometers, soapy cotton balls, small trash bag or waste can, running water, soaking basin with 70-percent alcohol, alcohol sponges or cotton balls, dry cotton balls or gauze pads, thermometer holder, disposable gloves

Procedure

1. Assemble equipment.
2. Wash hands. Put on gloves if needed.

   CAUTION: Follow standard precautions. Wear gloves if the thermometer was used for an oral or rectal temperature and was not covered with a plastic sheath.
3. After using the thermometer, use a soapy cotton ball or gauze pad to wipe the thermometer once from the top toward the tip or bulb (see figure 14-10A). Discard the soiled cotton ball in trash bag or waste can.

   NOTE: Rotate the thermometer while wiping it to clean all sides and parts.

4. With the bulb pointed downward, hold the thermometer by the stem and rinse the thermometer in cool water.

   CAUTION: Hot water will break the thermometer or destroy the mercury column.
5. Shake the thermometer down to 96°F (35.6°C) or lower.

   CAUTION: Hold the thermometer securely between your thumb and index finger. Use a snapping motion of the wrist. Avoid countertops, tables, and other surfaces.
6. Place the thermometer in a small basin or container filled with disinfectant solution (usually 70-percent alcohol). Make sure the thermometer is completely covered by the solution (see figure 14-10B).

   NOTE: Thirty minutes is usually the minimum time recommended for soaking.
7. Remove gloves and wash hands.
8. After 30 minutes, remove the thermometer from the soaking solution and use an alcohol

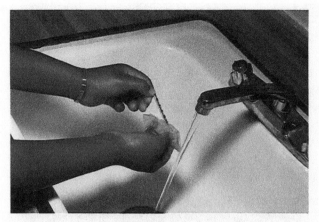

FIGURE 14-10A After each use, use a soapy cotton ball or gauze to wipe the thermometer in a circular motion from the stem to the bulb.

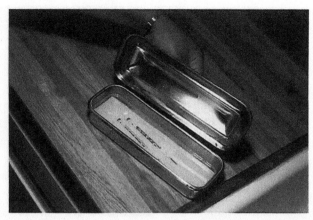

FIGURE 14-10B Soak the thermometer in a disinfectant solution for a minimum of 30 minutes.

cotton ball or alcohol sponge to wipe it from the stem toward the bulb. This removes any sediment from the thermometer.

9. Rinse the thermometer in cool water. Examine it carefully for any signs of breakage. Discard any broken thermometers according to the agency policy for disposal of mercury or mercury-containing items.

10. Read the thermometer to be sure it reads 96°F (35.6°C) or lower. Place it in a clean gauze-lined container. It is now ready for use.

    NOTE: Many health care agencies fill the container or thermometer holder with a disinfectant, usually 70-percent alcohol.

11. Replace all equipment used.

12. Remove gloves and discard in infectious container. Wash hands.

    NOTE: This procedure may vary according to agency policy.

Practice Go to the workbook and use the evaluation sheet for 14:2A, Cleaning a Clinical Thermometer, to practice this procedure. When you feel you have mastered this skill, sign the sheet and give it to your instructor for further action.

 Final Checkpoint Using the criteria listed on the evaluation sheet, your instructor will grade your performance.

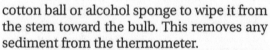

PROCEDURE 14:2B   OBRA
Measuring and Recording Oral Temperature

Equipment and Supplies

Oral thermometer, plastic sheath (if used), holder with disinfectant solution, tissues or dry cotton balls, container for used tissues, watch with second hand, soapy cotton balls, disposable gloves, notepaper, pencil/pen

Procedure

1. Assemble equipment.
2. Wash hands and put on gloves.

   CAUTION: Follow standard precautions for contact with saliva or the mucous membrane of the mouth.

3. Introduce yourself. Identify the patient. Explain the procedure.

4. Position the patient comfortably. Ask the patient if he/she has eaten, has had hot or cold fluids, or has smoked in the past 15 minutes.
   NOTE: Eating, drinking liquids, or smoking can affect the temperature in the mouth. Wait at least 15 minutes if the patient says "yes" to your question.

5. Remove the clean thermometer by the upper end. Use a clean tissue or dry cotton ball to wipe the thermometer from stem to bulb.
   NOTE: If the thermometer was soaking in a disinfectant, rinse first in cool water.
   ❗ CAUTION: Hold the thermometer securely to avoid breaking.

6. Read the thermometer to be sure it reads 96°F (35.6°C) or lower. Check carefully for chips or breaks.
   ❗ CAUTION: Never use a cracked thermometer because it may injure the patient.
   NOTE: If a plastic sheath is used, place it on the thermometer after checking for damage.

7. Insert the bulb under the patient's tongue, toward the side of the mouth (see figure 14-11). Ask the patient to hold it in place with the lips, and caution against biting it.
   NOTE: Check to be sure patient's mouth is closed.

8. Leave the thermometer in place for 3 to 5 minutes.
   NOTE: Some agencies require that the thermometer be left in place for 5 to 8 minutes. Follow your agency's policy.

9. Remove the thermometer. Hold it by the stem and use a tissue or cotton ball to wipe toward the bulb.
   NOTE: If a plastic sheath was used to cover the thermometer, there is no need to wipe the thermometer. Simply remove the sheath, taking care not to touch the part that was in the patient's mouth.
   ❗ CAUTION: Do *not* hold the bulb end. This could alter the reading because of the warmth of your hand.

10. Read the thermometer. Record the reading on notepaper.
    NOTE: Recheck the reading and your notation for accuracy.
    NOTE: If the reading is less than 97°F, reinsert the thermometer in the patient's mouth for 1 to 2 minutes.

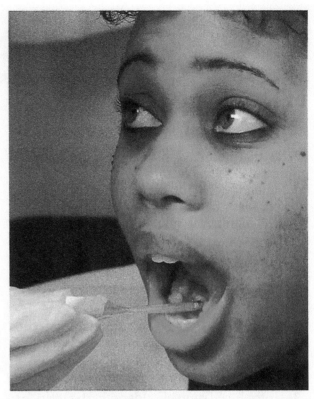

FIGURE 14-11 Insert the bulb of the thermometer under the patient's tongue (sublingually).

11. Clean the thermometer as instructed. Shake down to 96°F (35.6°C) or lower for next use.

12. Check the patient for comfort and safety before leaving.

13. Replace all equipment.

14. Remove gloves and discard in infectious waste container. Wash hands.

15. Record required information on the patient's chart or agency form, for example, date and time, T 98^6, your signature and title. Report any abnormal reading to your supervisor immediately.

Practice *Go to the workbook and use the evaluation sheet for 14:2B, Measuring and Recording Oral Temperature, to practice this procedure. When you feel you have mastered this skill, sign the sheet and give it to your instructor for further action.*

Final Checkpoint Using the criteria listed on the evaluation sheet, your instructor will grade your performance.

PROCEDURE 14:2C   OBRA

Measuring and Recording Rectal Temperature

Equipment and Supplies

Rectal thermometer, plastic sheath (if used), lubricant, tissues/cotton balls, waste bag or container, watch with second hand, paper, pencil/pen, soapy cotton ball, disposable gloves
NOTE: A manikin is frequently used to practice this procedure.

Procedure

1. Assemble equipment.
2. Wash hands and put on gloves.
   ⊛ CAUTION: Follow standard precautions if contact with rectal discharge is possible.
3. Introduce yourself. Identify the patient. Explain the procedure. Screen unit, draw curtains, and/or close door to provide privacy for the patient.
4. Remove rectal thermometer from its container. If the thermometer was soaking in a disinfectant, hold it by the stem end and rinse in cool water. Use a dry tissue/cotton ball to wipe from stem to bulb. Check that the thermometer reads 96°F (35.6°C) or lower. Check condition of thermometer. If a plastic sheath is used, position it on the thermometer.
   ❗ CAUTION: Breaks in a thermometer can injure the patient. Never use a cracked thermometer.
5. Place a small amount of lubricant on the tissue. Roll the bulb end of the thermometer in the lubricant to coat it. Leave the lubricated thermometer on the tissue until the patient is properly positioned.
6. Turn the patient on his or her side. If possible, use Sims' position (lying on left side with right leg bent up near the abdomen). Infants are usually placed on their backs, with legs raised and held securely, or on their abdomens (see figure 14-12).
7. Fold back covers just enough to expose the anal area.
   NOTE: Avoid exposing the patient unnecessarily.

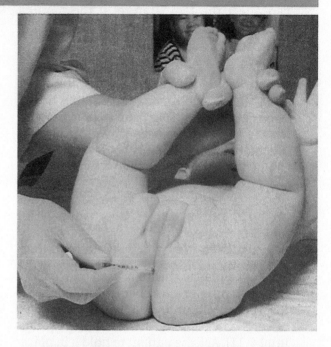

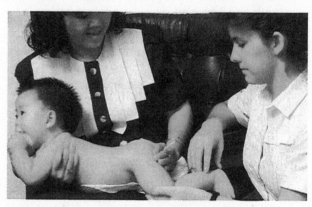

FIGURE 4-12 The infant can be positioned on the back or abdomen for a rectal temperature.

8. With one hand, raise the upper buttock gently. With the other hand, insert the lubricated thermometer approximately 1 to 1½ inches (½ to 1 inch for an infant) into the rectum. Tell the patient what you are doing.
   NOTE: At times, rotating the thermometer slightly will make it easier to insert.
   ❗ CAUTION: Never force the thermometer. It can break. If you are unable to insert it, obtain assistance.

9. Replace the covers. Keep your hand on the thermometer the entire time it is in place.

! **CAUTION:** *Never* let go of the thermometer. It could slide further into the rectum or break.

10. Hold the thermometer in place for 3 to 5 minutes.

11. Remove the thermometer gently. Tell the patient what you are doing.

12. Remove plastic sheath, if used, and discard it or use a tissue to remove excess lubricant from the thermometer. Wipe from stem to bulb. Hold by the stem area only. Discard the tissue into a waste container.

13. Read and record. Recheck your reading for accuracy. Remember to place an (R) next to the recording to indicate a rectal temperature was taken.

14. Reposition the patient. Observe all safety checkpoints before leaving the patient.

15. Clean the thermometer as instructed in Procedure 14:2A, Cleaning a Clinical Thermometer.

16. Replace all equipment.

17. Remove gloves and discard in infectious waste container. Wash hands.

18. **C** Record required information on the patient's chart or agency form, for example, date and time, T 99^6 (R), your signature and title. Report any abnormal reading immediately to your supervisor.

Practice *Go to the workbook and use the evaluation sheet for 14:2C, Measuring and Recording Rectal Temperature, to practice this procedure. When you feel you have mastered this skill, sign the sheet and give it to your instructor for further action.*

Final Checkpoint Using the criteria listed on the evaluation sheet, your instructor will grade your performance.

PROCEDURE 14:2D   OBRA

Measuring and Recording Axillary Temperature

Equipment and Supplies

Oral thermometer, plastic sheath (if used), disposable gloves (if needed), tissues/cotton balls, towel, waste container, watch with second hand, paper, pencil/pen, soapy cotton ball

Procedure

1. Assemble equipment.

2. Wash hands. Put on gloves if necessary.

 CAUTION: Follow standard precautions if contact with open sores or body fluids is possible.

3. Introduce yourself. Identify the patient. Explain the procedure.

4. Remove oral thermometer from its container. Use a tissue to wipe from stem to bulb. Check thermometer for damaged areas. Read the thermometer to be sure it reads below 96°F (36.5°C). Place a plastic sheath on the thermometer, if used.

5. Expose the axilla and use a towel to pat the armpit dry.

NOTE: Moisture can alter a temperature reading. Do not rub area hard because this too can alter the reading.

6. Raise the patient's arm and place the bulb end of the thermometer in the hollow of the axilla (see figure 14-13). Bring the arm over the chest and rest the hand on the opposite shoulder.

NOTE: This position holds the thermometer in place.

7. Leave the thermometer in place for 10 minutes.

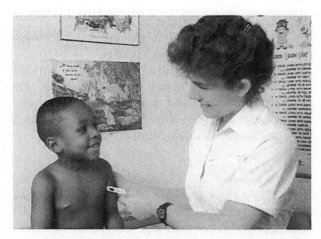

FIGURE 14-13 To take an axillary temperature, insert the bulb end of the thermometer in the hollow of the axilla or armpit.

8. Remove the thermometer. Remove sheath, if used, and discard. Wipe from stem to bulb to remove moisture. Hold by the stem end only.
   ! **CAUTION:** Holding the bulb end will change the reading.

9. Read and record. Check your reading for accuracy. Remember to mark (Ax) by the recording to indicate axillary temperature.

10. Reposition the patient. Be sure to check for safety and comfort before leaving.

11. Clean the thermometer as instructed.

12. Replace all equipment used.

13. Remove gloves and discard in an infectious waste container. Wash hands.

14. **C** Record required information on the patient's chart or agency form, for example, date and time, T 97^6 (Ax), your signature and title. Report any abnormal reading immediately to your supervisor.

Practice *Go to the workbook and use the evaluation sheet for 14:2D, Measuring and Recording Axillary Temperature, to practice this procedure. When you feel you have mastered this skill, sign the sheet and give it to your instructor for further action.*

Final Checkpoint Using the criteria listed on the evaluation sheet, your instructor will grade your performance.

PROCEDURE 14:2E   OBRA

Measuring and Recording Tympanic (Aural) Temperature

Equipment and Supplies

Tympanic thermometer, probe cover, paper, pencil/pen, container for soiled probe cover

Procedure

1. Assemble equipment.
   NOTE: Read the operating instructions so you understand exactly how the thermometer must be used.

2. Wash hands. Put on gloves if needed.
    CAUTION: Follow standard precautions if contact with open sores or body fluids is possible.

3. Introduce yourself. Identify the patient. Explain the procedure.

4. Remove the thermometer from its base. Set the thermometer on the proper mode according to operating instructions. The equal mode is usually used for newborn infants, the rectal mode for children under

3 years of age, and the oral mode for children over 3 years of age and all adults. In areas where core body temperatures are recorded, such as critical care units, the core mode may be used.

5. Install a probe cover according to instructions. This will usually activate the thermometer, showing the mode selected and the word *ready*, indicating the thermometer is ready for use.

   ! **CAUTION:** Do not use the thermometer until *ready* is displayed because inaccurate readings will result.

6. Position the patient. Infants under 1 year of age should be positioned lying flat with the head turned for easy access to the ear. Small children can be held on the parent's lap, with the head held against the parent's chest for support. Adults who can cooperate and hold the head steady can either sit or lie flat. Patients in bed should have the head turned to the side, and stabilized against the pillow.

7. Hold the thermometer in your right hand to take a temperature in the right ear, and in your left hand to take a temperature in the left ear. With your other hand, pull the ear pinna (external lobe) up and back on any child over 1 year of age and on adults. Pull the ear pinna straight back for infants under 1 year of age.

   NOTE: Pulling the pinna correctly straightens the auditory canal so the probe tip will point directly at the tympanic membrane.

8. Insert the covered probe into the ear canal as far as possible to seal the canal (see figure 14-14).

9. Hold the thermometer steady and press the scan or activation button. Hold it for the required amount of time, usually 1 to 2 seconds, until the reading is displayed on the screen.

10. Remove the thermometer from the patient's ear. Read and record the temperature. Place a (T) by the recording to indicate tympanic temperature.

    NOTE: The temperature will remain on the screen until the probe cover is removed.

    ! **CAUTION:** If the temperature reading is low or does not appear to be accurate,

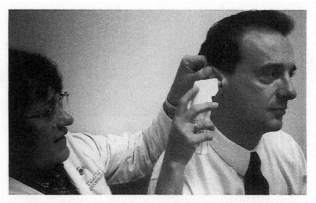

FIGURE 14-14 Insert the covered probe of the tympanic thermometer into the ear canal as far as possible to seal the canal.

change the probe cover and repeat the procedure. The opposite ear can be used for comparison.

11. Press the eject button on the thermometer to discard the probe cover into a waste container.

12. Return the thermometer to its base.

13. Reposition the patient. Observe all safety checkpoints before leaving the patient.

14. Remove gloves and discard in an infectious waste container. Wash hands.

15. **C** Record required information on the patient's chart or agency form, for example, date and time, T 98^0 (T), your signature and title. Report any abnormal reading immediately to your supervisor.

Practice *Go to the workbook and use the evaluation sheet for 14:2E, Measuring and Recording Tympanic (Aural) Temperature, to practice this procedure. When you feel you have mastered this skill, sign the sheet and give it to your instructor for further action.*

 Final Checkpoint Using the criteria listed on the evaluation sheet, your instructor will grade your performance.

PROCEDURE 14:2F

OBRA

Measuring Temperature with an Electronic Thermometer

Equipment and Supplies

Electronic thermometer with probe, sheath (probe cover), paper, pen/pencil, container for soiled sheath

Procedure

1. Assemble equipment.
   NOTE: Read the operating instructions for the electronic thermometer so you understand how the particular model operates.
2. Wash hands. Put on gloves.
   CAUTION: Follow standard precautions and wear gloves if you are taking a rectal or oral temperature.
3. Introduce yourself. Identify the patient. Explain the procedure.
4. Position the patient comfortably and correctly.
   NOTE: For an oral temperature, ask the patient if he/she has eaten, has had hot or cold fluids, or has smoked in the past 15 minutes. Wait at least 15 minutes if the patient answers "yes."
   NOTE: For a rectal temperature, position the patient in Sims' position if possible.
5. If the probe has to be connected to the thermometer unit, insert the probe into the correct receptacle. If the thermometer has an "on" or "activate" button, push the button to turn on the thermometer.
6. Cover the probe with the sheath or probe cover.
   NOTE: For a rectal temperature, the sheath must be lubricated.
7. Insert the covered probe into the desired location. Most probes are heavy, so it is usually necessary to hold the probe in position (see figure 14-15A).
   CAUTION: Hold on to the probe at all times for a rectal temperature.
8. When the unit signals that the temperature has been recorded, remove the probe.
   NOTE: Many electronic thermometers have an audible "beep." Others indicate that tem-

perature has been recorded when the numbers stop flashing and become stationary.
9. Read and record the temperature. Recheck your reading for accuracy.
   NOTE: Remember to place an (R) next to rectal readings or an (Ax) next to axillary readings.
10. Without touching the sheath or probe cover, remove it from the probe (see figure 14-15B). Many thermometers have a button you push to remove the sheath. Discard the sheath in an infectious waste container.
11. Reposition the patient. Observe all safety checkpoints before leaving the patient.
12. Return the probe to the correct storage position in the thermometer unit. Turn off the

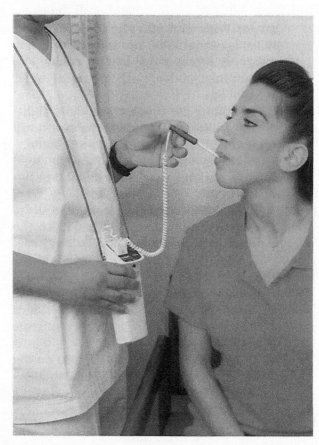

FIGURE 14-15A While taking a temperature, hold the probe of the electronic thermometer in place.

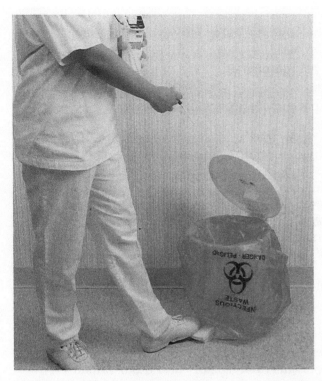

unit if this is necessary. Place the unit in the charging stand if the model has a charging unit.

13. Replace all equipment.

14. Remove gloves and discard in an infectious waste container. Wash hands.

15. **C** Record required information on the patient's chart or agency form, for example, date and time, T 98^8, your signature and title. Report any abnormal reading immediately to your supervisor.

FIGURE 14-15B Discard the probe cover in an infectious waste container without touching the cover.

Practice *Go to the workbook and use the evaluation sheet for 14:2F, Measuring Temperature with an Electronic Thermometer, to practice this procedure. When you feel you have mastered this skill, sign the sheet and give it to your instructor for further action.*

Final Checkpoint Using the criteria listed on the evaluation sheet, your instructor will grade your performance.

14:3 INFORMATION Measuring and Recording Pulse

OBRA Pulse is a vital sign that you will be required to take. There are certain facts you must know when you take this measurement. This section provides the main information.

Pulse is defined as "the pressure of the blood pushing against the wall of an artery as the heart beats and rests." In other words, it is a throbbing of the arteries that is caused by the contractions of the heart. The pulse is more easily felt in arteries that lie fairly close to the skin and can be pressed against a bone by the fingers.

The pulse can be felt at different arterial sites on the body. Some of the major sites are shown in figure 14-16 and include:

- temporal—at the side of the forehead
- carotid—at the neck
- brachial—inner aspect of forearm at the antecubital space (crease of the elbow)
- radial—at the inner aspect of the wrist, above the thumb
- femoral—at the inner aspect of the upper thigh
- popliteal—behind the knee
- dorsalis pedis—at the top of the foot arch

NOTE: Pulse is usually taken over the radial artery.

Pulse rate is measured as the number of beats per minute. Pulse rates vary among individuals, depending on age, sex, and body size:

- Adults have a general range of 60 to 90 beats per minute.
- Adult men: 60 to 70 beats per minute.
- Adult women: 65 to 80 beats per minute.

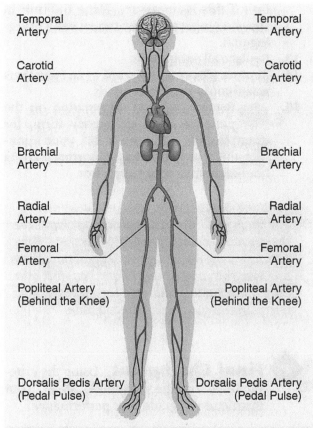

FIGURE 14-16 Major pulse sites.

- Children aged over 7: 70 to 90 beats per minute.
- Children aged from 1 to 7: range of 80 to 110 beats per minute.

- Infants: 100 to 160 beats per minute.
- **Bradycardia** is a pulse rate under 60 beats per minute.
- **Tachycardia** is a pulse rate over 100 beats per minute (except in children).

NOTE: Any variations or extremes in pulse rates should be reported immediately.

Rhythm of the pulse is also noted. Rhythm refers to the regularity of the pulse, or the spacing of the beats. It is described as *regular* or *irregular*. An **arrhythmia** is an irregular or abnormal rhythm, usually caused by a defect in the electrical conduction pattern of the heart.

Volume, or the strength or intensity of the pulse, is also noted. It is described by words such as *strong, weak, thready,* or *bounding.*

Various factors will change pulse rate. Increased, or accelerated, rates can be caused by exercise, stimulant drugs, excitement, fever, shock, nervous tension, and other similar factors. Decreased, or slower, rates can be caused by sleep, depressant drugs, heart disease, coma, physical training, and other similar factors.

STUDENT: *Go to the workbook and complete the assignment sheet for 14:3, Measuring and Recording Pulse. Then return and continue with the procedure.*

PROCEDURE 14:3   OBRA

Measuring and Recording Radial Pulse

Equipment and Supplies

Watch with second hand, paper, pencil/pen

Procedure

1. Assemble equipment.
2. Wash hands.
3. Introduce yourself. Identify the patient. Explain the procedure.

4. Place the patient in a comfortable position, with the arm supported and the palm of the hand turned downward.

   NOTE: If the forearm rests on the chest, it will be easier to count respirations after taking the pulse.

5. With the tips of your first two or three fingers, locate the pulse on the thumb side of the patient's wrist (see figure 14-17).

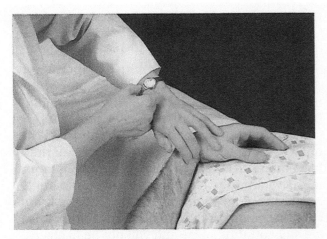

FIGURE 14-17 To count a radial pulse, put the tips of two or three fingers on the thumb side of the patient's wrist.

NOTE: Do not use your thumb; use your fingers. The thumb contains a pulse that you may confuse with the patient's pulse.

6. When the pulse is felt, exert slight pressure and start counting. Use the second hand of the watch and count for 1 full minute.

NOTE: In some agencies, the pulse is counted for 30 seconds and the final number multiplied by 2. To detect irregularities, it is better to count for 1 full minute.

7. While counting the pulse, also note the volume (character or strength) and the rhythm (regularity).

8. Record the following information: date, time, rate, rhythm, and volume. Follow your agency's policy for recording.

9. Check the patient before leaving. Observe all safety precautions to protect the patient.

10. Replace all equipment used.

11. Wash hands.

12. Record all required information on the patient's chart or agency form, for example, date, time, P 82 strong and regular, your signature and title. Report any unusual observations immediately to your supervisor.

Practice *Go to the workbook and use the evaluation sheet for 14:3, Measuring and Recording Radial Pulse, to practice this procedure. When you feel you have mastered this skill, sign the sheet and give it to your instructor for further action.*

Final Checkpoint Using the criteria listed on the evaluation sheet, your instructor will grade your performance.

14:4 INFORMATION Measuring and Recording Respirations

OBRA Respirations are another vital sign that you must observe, count, and record correctly. This section provides the main points you must note when counting and recording the quality of respirations.

Respiration is the process of taking in oxygen (O_2) and expelling carbon dioxide (CO_2) from the lungs and respiratory tract. One respiration consists of one inspiration (breathing in) and one expiration (breathing out).

The normal rate for respirations in adults is 14 to 18 breaths per minute, although wider ranges may be observed (12 to 20 breaths per minute). In children, respirations are slightly faster than those for adults and average 16 to 25 per minute. In infants, the rate may be 30 to 50 per minute.

In addition to rate, the character and rhythm of respirations should be noted. **Character** refers to the depth and quality of respirations. Words used to describe character include *deep, shallow, labored, difficult, stertorous* (abnormal sounds like snoring), and *moist*. Rhythm refers to the regularity of respirations, or equal spacing between breaths. It is described as *regular* or *irregular*.

The following terminology is used to describe abnormal respirations:

♦ **dyspnea**—difficult or labored breathing.

♦ **apnea**—absence of respirations, usually temporary.

- **tachypnea**—respiratory rate above 25 respirations per minute.
- **bradypnea**—slow respiratory rate, usually below 10 respirations per minute.
- **orthopnea**—severe dyspnea in which breathing is very difficult in any position other than sitting erect or standing.
- **Cheyne–Stokes** respirations—periods of dyspnea followed by periods of apnea; frequently noted in the dying patient.
- **rales**—bubbling or noisy sounds caused by fluids or mucus in the air passages.
- **wheezing**—difficult breathing with a high-pitched whistling or sighing sound during expiration; caused by a narrowing of bronchioles (as seen in asthma) and/or an obstruction or mucus accumulation in the bronchi.
- **cyanosis**—a dusky, bluish discoloration of the skin, lips, and/or nail beds as a result of decreased oxygen and increased carbon dioxide in the bloodstream.

Respirations must be counted in such a way that the patient is unaware of the procedure. Because respirations are partially under voluntary control, patients may breathe more quickly or more slowly when they become aware of the fact that respirations are being counted. Do not tell the patient you are counting respirations. Also, leave your hand on the pulse site while counting respirations. The patient will think you are still counting pulse and will not be likely to alter the respiratory rate.

STUDENT: *Go to the workbook and complete the assignment sheet for 14:4, Measuring and Recording Respirations. Then return and continue with the procedure.*

PROCEDURE 14:4　　OBRA

Measuring and Recording Respirations

Equipment and Supplies

Watch with second hand, paper, pen/pencil

Procedure

1. Assemble equipment.
2. Wash hands.
3. Introduce yourself. Identify the patient.
4. After the pulse rate has been counted, leave your hand in position on the pulse site and count the number of times the chest rises and falls during one minute (see figure 14-18).
   NOTE: This is done so the patient is not aware that respirations are being counted. If patients are aware, they can alter their rate of breathing.
5. Count each expiration and inspiration as one respiration.
6. Note the depth (character) and rhythm (regularity) of the respirations.

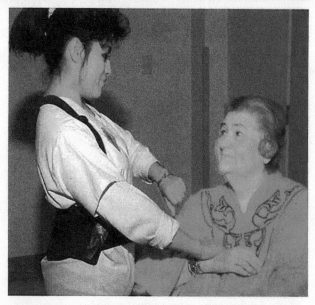

FIGURE 14-18 Positioning the patient's hand on his or her chest makes it easier to count pulse and respiration.

7. Record the following information: date, time, rate, character, and rhythm.
8. Check the patient before leaving the area. Observe all safety precautions to protect the patient.
9. Replace all equipment.
10. Wash hands.
11. Record all required information on the patient's chart or agency form, for example, date, time, R 16 deep and regular (or even), your signature and title. Report any unusual observations immediately to your supervisor.

Practice *Go to the workbook and use the evaluation sheet for 14:4, Measuring and Recording Respirations, to practice this procedure. When you feel you have mastered this skill, sign the sheet and give it to your instructor for further action.*

Final Checkpoint Using the criteria listed on the evaluation sheet, your instructor will grade your performance.

14:5 INFORMATION Graphing TPR

C In some agencies, you may be required to chart temperature, pulse, and respirations (TPR) on graphic records. This section provides basic information about these records.

Graphic sheets are special records used for recording temperature, pulse, and respirations. The forms vary in different health care facilities, but all contain the same basic information. The graphic chart presents a visual diagram of variations in a patient's vital signs. The progress is easier to follow than a list of numbers that give the same information. Graphic charts are used most often in hospitals and long-term-care facilities. However, similar records may be kept in medical offices or other health care facilities. Patients are sometimes taught how to maintain these records.

Some charts make use of color coding. For example, temperature is recorded in blue ink, pulse is recorded in red ink, and respirations are recorded in green ink. Other agencies use blue ink for 7 AM to 7 PM (days) and red ink for 7 PM to 7 AM (nights). Follow the policy of your institution.

Factors that affect vital signs are often included on the graph. Examples include surgery, medications that lower temperature (such as aspirin), and antibiotics.

The graph is a medical record, so it must be neat, legible, and accurate. Double check all information recorded on the graph. If an error occurs, it should be crossed out carefully with red ink and initialed. Correct information should then be inserted on the graph.

STUDENT: *Read the complete procedure for 14:5, Graphing TPR. Then go back and start doing the procedure. Your assignment will follow the procedure.*

PROCEDURE 14:5   C
Graphing TPR

Equipment and Supplies

Blank TPR graphic sheets in the workbook, TPR sample graph, assignment sheets on graphing in the workbook, pen, ruler

Procedure

1. Assemble equipment.
2. Examine the sample graphic sheet (see figure 14-19). This will vary, depending on the

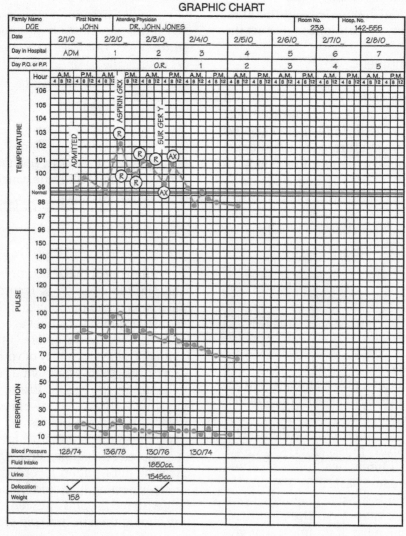

FIGURE 14-19 A sample graphic sheet.

agency. However, most graphic sheets contain time blocks across the top and number blocks for TPRs on the side. Note areas for recording temperature, pulse, and respirations. Refer to the example while completing the procedure steps.

3. Using a blank graphic sheet, fill in patient information in the spaces provided at the top. Write last name first in most cases. Be sure patient identification, hospital, and room number are accurate.

   NOTE: Forms vary. Follow directions as they apply to your form.

4. Fill in the dates in the spaces provided after DATE.

   NOTE: A graphic chart provides a day-to-day visual representation of the variations in a patient's TPRs.

5. If your chart calls for DAY IN HOSPITAL below the dates, enter *Adm.* under the first date. This stands for day of admission. The second date would then be day *1*, or first full day in the hospital. The third date would be day *2*, and so forth.

6. Some graphs contain a third line, DAYS P.O. or PP, which means days post-op (after surgery) or postpartum (after delivery of a baby). The day of surgery would be shown as *O.R.* or *Surgery*. The next day would be day *1*, or first day after surgery. The day of delivery of a baby is shown as *Del.*, with the next day as day *1*, or first day after delivery. Numbers continue in sequence for each following day.

7. Go to the Assignment Sheet #1. Note the TPRs. On the graphic sheet, find the correct

Date and Time column. Move down the column until the correct temperature number is found on the side of the chart. Mark this with a dot (•) in the box. Do the same for the pulse and respirations.

! CAUTION: Double check your notations. Be sure they are accurate.

✓ CHECKPOINT: Your instructor will check your notations.

8. Repeat step 7 for the next TPR. Check to be sure you are in the correct time column. Mark the dots clearly under the time column and at the correct temperature measurement, pulse rate, or respiration rate.

9. Use a straight paper edge or ruler to connect the dots for temperature. Do the same with the dots for pulse and, finally, with the dots for respiration.

NOTE: A ruler makes the line straight and neat, and the readings are more legible.

10. Continue to graph the remaining TPRs from Assignment Sheet #1. Double check all entries for accuracy. Use a ruler to connect all dots for each of the vital signs.

11. Any drug that might alter or change temperature or other vital signs is usually noted on the graph in the time column closest to the time when the drug was first given. Turn the paper sideways and write the name of the drug in the correct time column. Aspirin is often recorded in this column because it lowers temperature. A rapid drop in body temperature would be readily explained by the word *aspirin* in the time column. Antibiotics and medications that alter heart rate are also noted in many cases.

12. Other events in a patient's hospitalization are also recorded in the time column. Examples include surgery and discharge. In some hospitals, if the patient is placed in isolation, this is also noted on the graph.

13. Blood pressure, weight, height, defecation (bowel movements), and other similar kinds of information are often recorded in special areas at the bottom of the graphic record. Record any information required in the correct areas on your form.

14. Recheck your graph for neatness, accuracy, and completeness of information.

Practice *Go to the workbook and complete Assignment Sheet #1 for Graphing TPR. Give it to your instructor for grading. Note all changes. Then complete Assignment Sheet #2 for graphing TPR in the workbook. Repeat this process by completing Graphing TPR assignments #3 to #5 until you have mastered graphic records.*

 Final Checkpoint Your instructor will grade your performance on this skill according to the accuracy of the completed assignments.

14:6 INFORMATION Measuring and Recording Apical Pulse

At times, you will be required to take an apical pulse. This section provides basic information on this topic.

An **apical pulse** is a pulse count taken with a **stethoscope** at the apex of the heart. The actual heartbeat is heard and counted. A stethoscope is an instrument used to listen to internal body sounds. The stethoscope amplifies the sounds so they are easier to hear. Parts of the stethoscope include the earpieces, tubing, and bell or thin, flexible disk called a *diaphragm* (see figure 14-20). The tips of the earpieces should be bent forward when they are placed in the ears. The earpieces should fit snugly but should not cause pain or discomfort. To prevent the spread of microorganisms, the earpieces and bell/diaphragm of the stethoscope should be cleaned with a disinfectant such as alcohol before and after every use.

Usually, a physician orders an apical pulse. It is frequently ordered for patients with irregular heartbeats, hardening of the arteries, or weak or

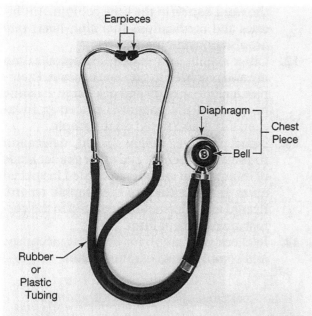

FIGURE 14-20 Parts of a stethoscope.

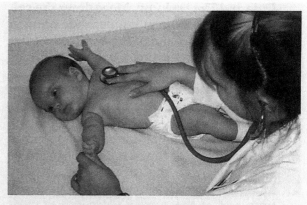

FIGURE 14-21 An apical pulse is frequently taken on infants and small children because their pulses are more rapid.

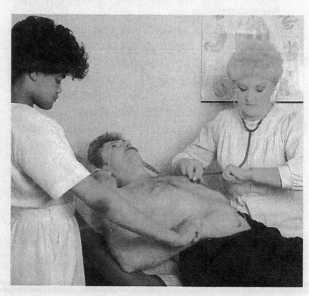

FIGURE 14-22 To determine a pulse deficit, one person should count an apical pulse while another person is counting a radial pulse.

rapid radial pulses. Because children and infants have very rapid radial pulse counts, apical pulse counts are usually taken (see figure 14-21). It is generally easier to count a rapid pulse while listening to it (through a stethoscope) than by feeling it with your fingers.

It is important that you protect the patient's privacy when counting an apical pulse. Avoid exposing the patient during this procedure.

Two separate heart sounds are heard while listening to the heartbeat. The sounds resemble a "lubb-dupp." Each lubb-dupp counts as one heartbeat. The sounds are caused by the closing of the heart valves as blood flows through the chambers of the heart. Any abnormal sounds or beats should be reported immediately to your supervisor.

A **pulse deficit** is a condition that occurs with some heart conditions. In some cases, the heart is weak and does not pump enough blood to produce a pulse. In other cases, the heart beats too fast (tachycardia), and there is not enough time for the heart to fill with blood; therefore, the heart does not produce a pulse during each beat. In such cases, the apical pulse rate is higher than the pulse rate at other pulse sites on the body. For the most accurate determination of a pulse deficit, one person should check the apical pulse while a second person checks another pulse site, usually the radial pulse (see figure 14-22). If this is not possible, one person should first check the apical pulse and then immediately check the radial pulse. Then, subtract the rate of the radial pulse from the rate of the apical pulse. The difference is the pulse deficit. For example, if the apical pulse is 130 and the radial pulse is 92, the pulse deficit would be 38 (130 − 92 = 38).

STUDENT: *Go to the workbook and complete the assignment sheet for 14:6, Measuring and Recording Apical Pulse. Then return and continue with the procedure.*

PROCEDURE 14:6

Measuring and Recording Apical Pulse

Equipment and Supplies

Stethoscope, watch with second hand, paper, pencil/pen, alcohol or disinfectant swab

Procedure

1. Assemble equipment. Use alcohol or a disinfectant to wipe the earpieces and the bell/diaphragm of the stethoscope.
2. Wash hands.
3. Introduce yourself. Identify the patient and explain the procedure. If the patient is an infant or child, explain the procedure to the parent(s).

    NOTE: It is usually best to say, "I am going to listen to your heartbeat." Some patients do not know what an apical pulse is.
4. Close the door to the room. Screen the unit or draw curtains around the bed to provide privacy.
5. Uncover the left side of the patient's chest. The stethoscope must be placed directly against the skin.
6. Place the stethoscope tips in your ears. Locate the apex of the heart, 2 to 3 inches to the left of the breastbone. Use your index finger to locate the fifth intercostal (between the ribs) space at the midclavicular (collarbone) line (see figure 14-23). Place the bell/diaphragm over the apical region and listen for heart sounds.

    ⓘ CAUTION: Be sure the tips of the stethoscope are facing forward before placing them in your ears.
7. Count the apical pulse for 1 full minute. Note the rate, rhythm, and volume.

    NOTE: Remember to count each lubb-dupp as one beat.
8. If you doubt your count, recheck your count for another minute.
9. Record your reading. Note date, time, rate, rhythm, and volume. Chart according to the agency policy. Some use an A and others use an AP to denote apical pulse.

    NOTE: If both a radial and apical pulse are taken, it may be recorded as A82/R82. If a pulse deficit exists, it should be noted. For example, with A80/R64, there

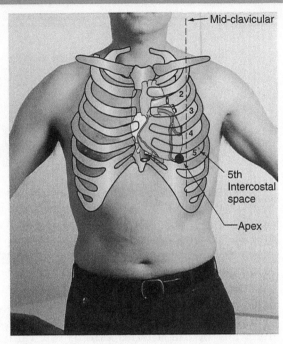

FIGURE 14-23 Locate the apex of the heart at the fifth intercostal (between the ribs) space by the midclavicular (middle of the collarbone) line.

is a pulse deficit of 16 (that is, 80 − 64 = 16). This would be recorded as A80/R64 Pulse deficit: 16.

10. Check all safety and comfort points before leaving the patient.
11. Use an alcohol or disinfectant swab to clean the earpieces and the bell/diaphragm of the stethoscope. Replace all equipment.
12. Wash hands.
13. ⓒ Record all required information on the patient's chart or agency form. For example: date, time, AP 86 strong and regular, your signature and title. If any abnormalities or changes were observed, note and report these immediately.

Practice *Go to the workbook and use the evaluation sheet for 14:6, Measuring and Recording Apical Pulse, to practice this procedure. When you feel you have mastered this skill, sign the sheet and give it to your instructor for further action.*

Final Checkpoint Using the criteria listed on the evaluation sheet, your instructor will grade your performance.

14:7 INFORMATION Measuring and Recording Blood Pressure

OBRA Blood pressure (BP) is one of the vital signs you will be required to take. It is important that your recording be accurate and that you understand what the blood pressure reading means. This section provides basic information on this topic.

Blood pressure (BP) is a measurement of the pressure that the blood exerts on the walls of the arteries during the various stages of heart activity. Blood pressure is read in millimeters (mm) of mercury (Hg) on an instrument known as a **sphygmomanometer.**

There are two types of blood pressure measurements: systolic and diastolic. **Systolic** pressure occurs in the walls of the arteries when the left ventricle of the heart is contracting and pushing blood into the arteries.

◆ A normal systolic reading is 120 millimeters mercury (120 mm Hg).

◆ Normal range for systolic readings is from 100 to 140 mm Hg.

Diastolic pressure is the constant pressure in the walls of the arteries when the left ventricle of the heart is at rest, or between contractions. Blood has moved forward into the capillaries and veins, so the volume of blood in the arteries has decreased.

◆ A normal diastolic reading is 80 mm Hg.

◆ Normal range for diastolic readings is from 60 to 90 mm Hg.

Pulse pressure is the difference between systolic and diastolic pressure. The pulse pressure is an important indicator of the health and tone of arterial walls. A normal range for pulse pressure in adults is 30 to 50 mm Hg. For example, if the systolic pressure is 120 mm Hg and the diastolic pressure is 80 mm Hg, the pulse pressure is 40 mm Hg (120 minus 80 = 40).

Hypertension, or high blood pressure, is indicated when pressures are greater than 140 mm Hg systolic and 90 mm Hg diastolic. Common causes include stress, anxiety, obesity, high-salt intake, aging, kidney disease, thyroid deficiency, and vascular conditions such as arteriosclerosis. If hypertension is not treated, it can lead to stroke, kidney disease, and/or heart disease.

Hypotension, or low blood pressure, is indicated when pressures are less than 100 mm Hg systolic and 60 mm Hg diastolic. Hypotension may occur with heart failure, dehydration, depression, severe burns, hemorrhage, and shock. *Orthostatic*, or postural, hypotension occurs when there is a sudden drop in both systolic and diastolic pressure when an individual moves from a lying to a sitting or standing position. It is caused by the inability of blood vessels to compensate quickly to the change in position. The individual becomes lightheaded and dizzy and may experience blurred vision. The symptoms last a few seconds until the blood vessels compensate and more blood is pushed to the brain.

Various factors can influence blood pressure readings. Some of these factors are:

◆ force of the heartbeat

◆ resistance of the arterial system

◆ elasticity of the arteries

◆ volume of the blood in the arteries

Many other factors can also influence blood pressure readings. These factors can cause blood pressure to be high or low. Some examples are as follows:

◆ factors that may increase blood pressure:
  (1) excitement, anxiety, nervous tension
  (2) stimulant drugs

(3) exercise and eating
(4) smoking

◆ factors that may decrease blood pressure:
(1) rest or sleep
(2) depressant drugs
(3) shock
(4) excessive loss of blood
(5) fasting (not eating)

◆ factors that may cause changes in readings:
(1) lying down
(2) sitting position
(3) standing position

Blood pressure is recorded as a fraction. The systolic reading is the top number, or numerator. The diastolic reading is the bottom number, or denominator. For example, a systolic reading of 120 and a diastolic reading of 80 is recorded as 120/80.

Two main types of sphygmomanometers are used to obtain blood pressure readings. The mercury sphygmomanometer has a long column of mercury (see figure 14-24). Each mark on the gauge represents 2 mm Hg. The mercury sphygmomanometer must always be placed on a flat, level surface or mounted on a wall. If it is calibrated correctly, the level of mercury should be at zero when viewed at eye level. The Occupational Health and Safety Administration (OSHA) discourages the use of mercury sphygmomanometers because of the possibility of a mercury spill and contamination. The aneroid sphygmomanometer does not have a mercury column (see figure 14-25). However, it is calibrated in mm Hg. Each line represents 2 mm Hg pressure. When the cuff is deflated, the needle must be on zero. If the needle is not on zero, the sphygmomanometer should not be used until it is recalibrated. Electronic sphygmomanometers are used in some health care facilities (see figure 14-26). Blood pressure and pulse readings are shown on a digital display after a cuff is placed on the patient.

In order to obtain accurate blood pressure readings, it is important to observe several factors. The American Heart Association (AHA) recommends that the patient sit quietly for at least 5 minutes before blood pressure is taken. The AHA also recommends that two separate readings be taken and averaged, with a minimum wait of 30 seconds between readings.

The size and placement of the sphygmomanometer cuff is also important (see figure 14-27). The cuff contains a rubber bladder that fills with air to apply pressure to the arteries. Cuffs that are too wide or too narrow give inaccurate readings. A cuff that is too small will give an artificially high reading; if it is too large it will give an artificially low reading. To ensure the greatest degree of accuracy, the width of the cuff should be approximately 20 percent wider than the diameter (or width) of the patient's upper arm. The patient should be seated or lying comfortably and have the forearm supported on a flat surface. The area of the arm covered by the cuff should be at heart level. The arm must be

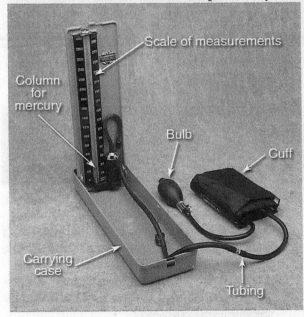

FIGURE 14-24 The gauge on a mercury sphygmomanometer has a column of mercury.

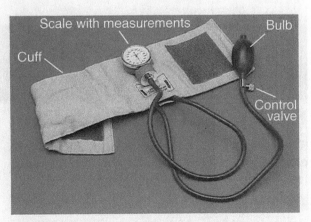

FIGURE 14-25 The gauge on an aneroid sphygmomanometer does not contain a column of mercury.

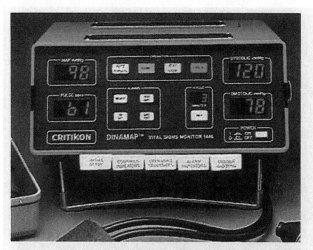

FIGURE 14-26 Electronic sphygmomanometers provide a digital display of blood pressure and pulse readings.

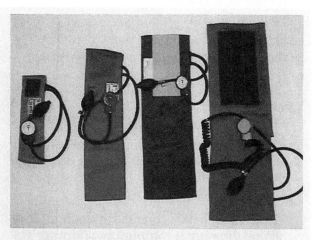

FIGURE 14-27 It is important to use the correct size cuff because cuffs that are too wide or too narrow will result in inaccurate readings.

free of any constrictive clothing. The deflated cuff should be placed on the arm with the center of the bladder in the cuff directly over the brachial artery, and the lower edge of the cuff 1 to 1½ inches above the antecubital area (bend of the elbow).

A final point relating to accuracy is placement of the stethoscope bell/diaphragm. The bell/diaphragm should be placed directly over the brachial artery at the antecubital area and held securely but with as little pressure as possible.

C For a health care worker, a major responsibility is accuracy in taking and recording

blood pressure. You should *not* discuss the reading with the patient. This is the responsibility of the physician because the information may cause a personal reaction that can affect the treatment. Only the physician should determine whether an abnormal blood pressure is indication for treatment.

STUDENT: *Go to the workbook and complete the assignment sheets for 14:7, Measuring and Recording Blood Pressure, Reading a Mercury Sphygmomanometer, and Reading an Aneroid Sphygmomanometer. Then return and continue with the procedure.*

PROCEDURE 14:7   OBRA

Measuring and Recording Blood Pressure

Equipment and Supplies

Stethoscope, sphygmomanometer, alcohol swab or disinfectant, paper, pencil/pen

Procedure

1. Assemble equipment. Use an alcohol swab or disinfectant to clean the earpieces and bell/diaphragm of the stethoscope.
2. Wash hands.

3. Introduce yourself. Identify the patient. Explain the procedure.
   NOTE: If possible, allow the patient to sit quietly for 5 minutes before taking the blood pressure.
   NOTE: Reassure the patient as needed. Nervous tension and excitement can alter or elevate blood pressure.
4. Roll up the patient's sleeve to approximately 5 inches above the elbow. Position the arm so that it is supported, comfortable, and

close to the level of the heart. The palm should be up.

NOTE: If the sleeve constricts the arm, remove the garment. The arm must be bare and unconstricted for an accurate reading.

5. Wrap the deflated cuff around the upper arm 1 to 1½ inches above the elbow and over the brachial artery. The center of the bladder inside the cuff should be over the brachial artery.

   CAUTION: Do not pull the cuff too tight. The cuff should be smooth and even.

6. Determine the palpatory systolic pressure (see figure 14-28A). To do this, find the radial pulse and keep your fingers on it. Inflate the cuff until the radial pulse disappears. Inflate the cuff 30 mm Hg above this point. Slowly release the pressure on the cuff while watching the gauge. When the pulse is felt again, note the reading on the gauge. This is the palpatory systolic pressure.

7. Deflate the cuff completely. Ask the patient to raise the arm and flex the fingers to promote blood flow. Wait 30 to 60 seconds to allow blood flow to resume completely.

8. Use your fingertips to locate the brachial artery (see figure 14-28B). The brachial artery is located on the inner part of the arm at the antecubital space (area where the elbow bends). Place the stethoscope over the artery (see figure 14-28C). Put the earpieces in your ears.

NOTE: Earpieces should be pointed forward.

9. Check to make sure the tubings are separate and not tangled together.

10. Gently close the valve on the rubber bulb by turning it in a clockwise direction. Inflate the cuff to 30 mm Hg above the palpatory systolic pressure.

    NOTE: Make sure the sphygmomanometer gauge is at eye level.

11. Open the bulb valve slowly and let the air escape gradually.

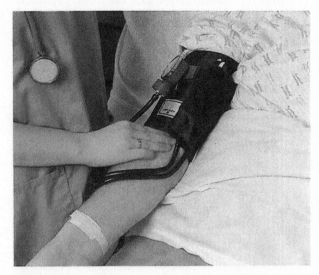

FIGURE 14-28B Locate the brachial artery on the inner part of the arm at the antecubital space.

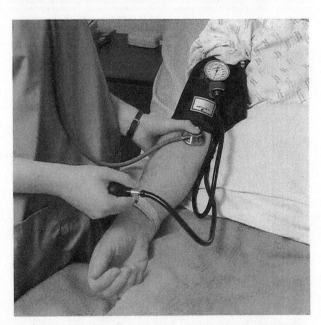

FIGURE 14-28C Place the stethoscope over the brachial artery as you listen for the blood pressure sounds.

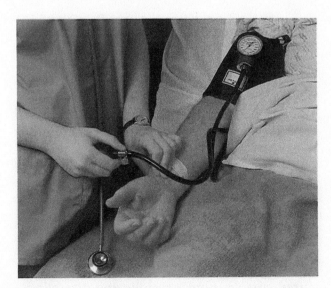

FIGURE 14-28A Determine the palpatory systolic pressure by checking the radial pulse as you inflate the cuff.

12. When the first sound is heard, note the reading on the manometer. This is the systolic pressure.

13. Continue to release the air until there is an abrupt change of the sound, usually soft or muffled. Note the reading on the manometer. Continue to release the air until the sound changes again, becoming first faint and then no longer heard. Note the reading on the manometer. The point at which the first change in sound occurs is the diastolic pressure in children. The diastolic pressure in adults is the point at which the sound becomes very faint or stops.

    NOTE: If you still hear sound, continue to the zero mark. Record both readings (the change of sound and the zero reading). For a systolic of 122 and a continued diastolic of 78, this can be written as 122/78/0.

14. When the sound ceases, rapidly deflate the cuff.

15. If you need to repeat the procedure to recheck your reading, completely deflate the cuff, wait 1 minute, and repeat the procedure. Ask the patient to raise the arm and flex the fingers to promote blood flow.

    ⚠ CAUTION: If you cannot obtain a reading, report to your supervisor promptly.

16. Record the time and your reading. The reading is written as a fraction, with systolic over diastolic. For example, BP 124/72 (or 124/80/72 if the change in sound is noted).

17. Remove the cuff. Expel any remaining air by squeezing the cuff. Use alcohol or a disinfectant to clean the stethoscope earpieces and diaphragm/bell. Replace all equipment.

18. Check patient for safety and comfort before leaving.

19. Wash hands.

20. Record all required information on the patient's chart or agency form, for example, date, time, B. P. 126/74, your signature and title. Report any abnormal readings immediately to your supervisor.

> **Practice** *Go to the workbook and use the evaluation sheet for 14:7, Measuring and Recording Blood Pressure, to practice this procedure. When you feel you have mastered this skill, sign the sheet and give it to your instructor for further action.*

✔ **Final Checkpoint** Using the criteria listed on the evaluation sheet, your instructor will grade your performance.

UNIT 14 SUMMARY

Vital signs are important indicators of health states of the body. The four main vital signs are temperature, pulse, respiration, and blood pressure.

Temperature is a measurement of the balance between heat lost and heat produced by the body. It can be measured orally, rectally, aurally (by way of the ear), and between folds of skin. An abnormal body temperature can indicate disease.

Pulse is the pressure of the blood felt against the wall of an artery as the heart contracts or beats. Pulse can be measured at various body sites, but the most common site is the radial pulse, which is at the wrist. The rate, rhythm, and volume (strength) should be noted each time a pulse is taken. An apical pulse is taken with a stethoscope at the apex of the heart. The stethoscope is used to listen to the heart beat. Apical pulse is frequently taken on infants and small children with rapid pulse rates.

Respiration refers to the breathing process. Each respiration consists of an inspiration (breathing in) and an expiration (breathing out). The rate, rhythm, and character, or type, of respirations should always be noted.

Blood pressure is the force exerted by the blood against the arterial walls when the heart contracts or relaxes. Two measurements are noted: systolic and diastolic. An abnormal blood pressure can indicate disease.

Vital signs are major indications of body function. The health care worker must use precise methods to measure vital signs so results are as accurate as possible. A thorough understanding of vital signs and what they indicate will allow the health care worker to be alert to any abnormalities so they can be immediately reported to the correct individual.

INTERNET SEARCHES

Use the suggested search engines in Unit 11:4 of this textbook to search the Internet for additional information on the following topics:

1. *Organization:* find the American Heart Association web site to obtain information on the heart, pulse, arrhythmias, and blood pressure.

2. *Vital signs:* research body temperature, pulse, respiration, blood pressure, and apical pulse.

3. *Temperature scales:* research Celcius (Centigrade) versus Fahrenheit temperatures. Try to locate conversion charts which can be used to compare the two scales.

4. *Diseases:* research hypothermia, fever or pyrexia, hypertension, hypotension, and heart arrhythmias.

REVIEW QUESTIONS

1. List the four (4) main vital signs.

2. State the normal value or range for an adult for each of the following:
   a. oral temperature
   b. rectal temperature
   c. axillary or groin temperature
   d. pulse
   e. respiration

3. What three (3) factors must be noted about every pulse?

4. Why is an apical pulse taken?

5. What is the pulse deficit if an apical pulse is 112 and the radial pulse is 88?

6. Differentiate between hypertension and hypotension and list the basic causes of each.

7. How does systolic pressure differ from diastolic pressure? What are the normal ranges for each?

8. Define each of the following:
   a. bradycardia
   b. arrhythmia
   c. dyspnea
   d. tachypnea
   e. rales

UNIT 14

SUGGESTED REFERENCES

American Heart Association. *Hypertension Primer.* 2nd ed. Dallas, TX: American Heart Association, 1999.

American Heart Association. *Recommendations for Human Blood Pressure Determination by Sphygmomanometers.* Dallas, TX: American Heart Association, n.d.

Cohen, Barbara, and Dena Wood. *Memmler's Structure and Function of the Human Body.* 7th ed. Philadelphia, PA: Lippincott, Williams, & Wilkins, 2000.

Hegner, Barbara, Esther Caldwell, and Joan Needham. *Nursing Assistant: A Nursing Process Approach.* 8th ed. Clifton Park, NY: Delmar Learning, 1999.

Huber, Helen, and Audree Spatz. *Homemaker– Home Health Aide.* 5th ed. Clifton Park, NY: Delmar Learning, 1998.

Keir, Lucille, Connie Krebs, and Barbara A. Wise. *Medical Assisting: Clinical and Administrative Competencies.* 5th ed. Clifton Park, NY: Delmar Learning, 2003.

Phipps, Wilma, Judith Sands, and Jane Marek. *Medical Surgical Nursing: Concepts and Clinical Practice.* St. Louis, MO: C. V. Mosby, 1998.

Simmers, Louise. *Practical Problems in Mathematics for Health Occupations.* Clifton Park, NY: Delmar Learning, 1996.

Zakus, Sharron. *Clinical Skills for Medical Assistants.* 4th ed. St. Louis, MO: C. V. Mosby, 2001.

CHAPTER 4

First Aid

Chapter Objectives

After completing this chapter,
you should be able to:

◆ Demonstrate cardiopulmonary resuscitation
for one-person rescue, two-person rescue,
infants, children, and obstructed-airway
victims

◆ Describe first aid for
—bleeding and wounds
—shock
—poisoning
—burns
—heat exposure
—cold exposure
—bone and joint injuries, including fractures
—specific injuries to the eyes, head, nose, ears,
chest, abdomen, and genital organs
—sudden illness including heart attack, stroke,
fainting, convulsions, and diabetic reactions

◆ Apply dressings and bandages, observing all
safety precautions and using the circular,
spiral, figure-eight, and recurrent, or finger
wrap

◆ Define, pronounce, and spell all key terms

Observe Standard
Precautions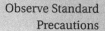

Instructor's Check—Call
Instructor at This Point

Safety—Proceed with
Caution

OBRA Requirement—Based
on Federal Law

Math Skill

Legal Responsibility

Science Skill

Career Information

Communications Skill

Technology

KEY TERMS

abrasion *(ah"-bray'-shun)*
amputation
avulsion *(ay"-vul'-shun)*
bandages
burn
cardiopulmonary
   resuscitation *(car'-dee-oh-*
   pull'-meh-nah-ree ree"-
   suh-sih-tay'-shun)
cerebrovascular accident
   (seh-ree'-bro-vass"-ku-lehr
   ax'-ih-dent)
convulsion
diabetic coma

diaphoresis
   (dy"-ah-feh-ree'-sis)
dislocation
dressing
fainting
first aid
fracture
frostbite
heart attack
heat cramps
heat exhaustion
heat stroke
hemorrhage

hypothermia
incision
infection
insulin shock
laceration
poisoning
puncture
shock
sprain
strain
triage *(tree'-ahj)*
wound

16:1 INFORMATION

Providing First Aid

INTRODUCTION

In every health care career you may have experiences that require a knowledge of first aid. This section provides basic guidelines for all the first aid topics discussed in the remaining sections of this unit. All students are strongly encouraged to take the First Aid Certification Course through their local Red Cross divisions to become proficient in providing first aid.

First aid is not full and complete treatment. Rather, **first aid** is best defined as "immediate care that is given to the victim of an injury or illness to minimize the effect of the injury or illness until experts can take over." Application of correct first aid can often mean the difference between life and death, or recovery versus permanent disability. In addition, by knowing the proper first aid measures, you can help yourself and others in a time of emergency.

BASIC PRINCIPLES OF FIRST AID

In any situation where first aid treatment is necessary, it is essential that you remain calm. Avoid panic. Evaluate the situation thoroughly. Always have a reason for anything you do. The treatment you provide will vary depending on the type of injury or illness, the environment, others present, equipment or supplies on hand, and the availability of medical help. Therefore, it is important for you to think about all these factors and determine what action is necessary.

The first step of first aid is to recognize that an emergency exists. Many senses can alert you to an emergency. Listen for unusual sounds such as screams, calls for help, breaking glass, screeching tires, or changes in machinery or equipment noises. Look for unusual sights such as an empty medicine container, damaged electrical wires, a stalled car, smoke or fire, a person lying motionless, blood, or spilled chemicals. Note any unusual, unfamiliar, or strange odors such as those of chemicals, natural gas, or pungent fumes. Watch for unusual appearances or behaviors in others such as difficulty in breathing, clutching of the chest or throat, abnormal skin colors, slurred or confused speech, unexplained confusion or drowsiness, excessive perspiration, signs of pain, and any symptoms of distress. Sometimes, signs of an emergency are clearly evident. An example is an automobile accident with victims in cars or on the street. Other times, signs are less obvious and require an alert individual to note that something is different or wrong. An empty medicine container and a small child with slurred speech, for example, are less obvious signs.

After determining that an emergency exists, the next step is to take appropriate action to help the victim or victims. Check the scene and make sure it is safe to approach. A quick glance at the area can provide information on what has occurred, dangers present, number of people involved, and other important factors. If live electrical wires are lying on the ground around an accident victim, for example, a rescuer could be electrocuted while trying to assist the victim. An infant thrown from a car during an automobile accident may be overlooked. A rescuer who pauses briefly to assess the situation will avoid such dangerous pitfalls and provide more efficient care. If the scene is not safe, call for medical help. Do not endanger your own life or the lives of other bystanders. Allow professionals to handle fires, dangerous chemicals, damaged electrical wires, and other life-threatening situations.

If the scene appears safe, approach the victim. Determine whether the victim is conscious (figure 16-1). If the victim shows no sign of consciousness, tap him gently and call to him. If the victim shows signs of consciousness, try to find out what happened and what is wrong. Never move an injured victim unless the victim is in a dangerous area such as an area filled with fire and/or smoke, flood waters, or carbon monoxide or poisonous fumes, or one with dangerous traffic, where vehicles cannot be stopped. If it is necessary to move the victim, do so as quickly and carefully as possible. Victims have been injured more severely by improper movement at the scenes of accidents, so avoid any unnecessary movement.

In an emergency, it is essential to call the emergency medical services (EMS) as soon as possible (figure 16-2). The time factor is critical. Early access to the EMS system and advanced medical care increases the victim's chance of survival. Use a telephone, cellular phone, or CB radio to contact the police, ambulance or rescue squad, fire department, utility company, or other resources. In most areas of the country, the emergency number 911 can be used to contact any of the emergency medical services. Sometimes, it may be necessary to instruct others to contact authorities while you are giving first aid. Make sure that complete, accurate information is given to the correct authority. Describe the situation, actions taken, exact location, telephone number from which you are calling, assistance required, number of people involved, and the condition of the victim(s). Do not hang up the receiver or end the CB radio call until the other party has all the necessary information. If you are alone, call EMS immediately before providing any care to:

♦ an unconscious adult

♦ an unconscious child who has reached puberty

♦ an unconscious infant or child with a high risk for heart problems

♦ any victim for whom you witness a sudden cardiac arrest

If you are alone, shout for help and start cardiopulmonary resuscitation (CPR) if needed for:

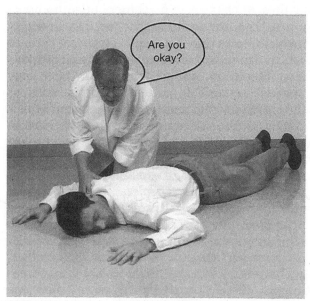

FIGURE 16-1 Determine whether the victim is conscious by gently tapping and by calling to him or her.

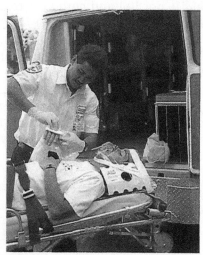

FIGURE 16-2 Call for emergency medical services (EMS) as soon as possible.

- an unconscious infant or child 1 year of age to puberty
- any victim of submersion or near drowning
- any victim with cardiac arrest caused by a drug overdose or trauma

If no one arrives to call EMS, continue providing care by giving five cycles of CPR (approximately 2 minutes). Then go to the nearest telephone, call for EMS, and return immediately to the victim.

After calling for help, provide care to the victim. If possible, obtain the victim's permission before providing any care. Introduce yourself and ask if you can help. If the victim can respond, he or she should give you permission before you provide care. If the victim is a child or minor, and a parent is present, obtain permission from the parent. If the victim is unconscious, confused, or seriously ill and unable to consent to care, and no other relative is available to give permission, you can assume that you have permission. It is important to remember that every individual has the right to refuse care. If a person refuses to give consent for care, do not proceed. If possible, have someone witness the refusal of care. If a life-threatening emergency exists, call EMS, alert them to the situation, and allow the professionals to take over.

At times it may be necessary to **triage** the situation. Triage is a method of prioritizing treatment. If a victim has more than one injury or illness, the most severe injury or illness must be treated first. If two or more people are involved, triage also determines which person is treated first. Life-threatening emergencies must be treated first. Examples include:

- no breathing or difficulty in breathing
- no pulse
- severe bleeding
- persistent pain in the chest or abdomen
- vomiting or passing blood
- poisoning
- head, neck, or spine injuries
- open chest or abdominal wounds
- shock
- severe partial-thickness and all full-thickness burns

Proper care for these emergencies is described in the sections that follow. If the victim is con-scious, breathing, and able to talk, reassure the victim and try to determine what has happened. Examine the victim thoroughly. Always have a sound reason for anything you do. Examples include:

- Ask the victim about pain or discomfort
- Check the victim for other types of injuries such as fractures (broken bones), burns, shock, and specific injuries
- Note any abnormal signs or symptoms
- Check vital signs
- Note the temperature, color, and moistness of the skin
- Check and compare the pupils of the eyes
- Look for fluids or blood draining from the mouth, nose, or ears
- Gently examine the body for cuts, bruises, swelling, and painful areas

Report any abnormalities noted to emergency medical services when they arrive at the scene.

Obtain as much information regarding the accident, injury, or illness as possible. This information can then be given to the correct authorities. Information can be obtained from the victim, other persons present, or by examination of items present at the scene. Emergency medical identification contained in a bracelet, necklace, medical card, or Vial-of-Life is an important source of information. Empty medicine containers, bottles of chemicals or solutions, or similar items also can reveal important information. Be alert to all such sources of information. Use this information to determine how you may help the victim.

SUMMARY

Some general principles of care should be observed whenever first aid is necessary. Some of these principles are:

- Obtain qualified assistance as soon as possible. Report all information obtained, observations noted, treatment given, and other important facts to the correct authorities. It may sometimes be necessary to send someone at the scene to obtain help.
- Avoid any unnecessary movement of the victim. Keep the victim in a position that will

allow for providing the best care for the type of injury or illness.

♦ Reassure the victim. A confident, calm attitude will help relieve the victim's anxiety.

♦ If the victim is unconscious or vomiting, do not give him or her anything to eat or drink. It is best to avoid giving a victim anything to eat or drink while providing first aid treatment, unless the specific treatment requires that fluids or food be given.

♦ Protect the victim from cold or chilling, but avoid overheating the victim.

♦ Work quickly, but in an organized and efficient manner.

♦ Do not make a diagnosis or discuss the victim's condition with observers at the scene. It is essential to maintain confidentiality and protect the victim's right to privacy while providing treatment.

♦ Make every attempt to avoid further injury.

CAUTION: Provide only the treatment that you are qualified to provide.

STUDENT: *Go to the workbook and complete the assignment sheet for 16:1, Providing First Aid.*

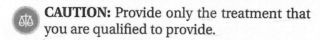

16:2 INFORMATION

Performing Cardiopulmonary Resuscitation

INTRODUCTION

At some time in your life, you may find an unconscious victim who is not breathing. This is an emergency situation. Correct action can save a life. Students are strongly encouraged to take certification courses in cardiopulmonary resuscitation (CPR) offered by the American Red Cross and American Heart Association. This section provides the basic facts about CPR for health care providers according to the 2005 American Heart Association standards. *The information provided is not intended to take the place of an approved certification course.*

The word parts of **cardiopulmonary resuscitation** provide a fairly clear description of the procedure: cardio (the heart) plus pulmonary (the lungs) plus resuscitation (to remove from apparent death or unconsciousness). When you administer CPR, you breathe for the person *and* circulate the blood. The purpose is to keep oxygenated blood flowing to the brain and other vital body organs until the heart and lungs start working again, or until medical help is available.

Clinical death occurs when the heart stops beating and the victim stops breathing. *Biological death* refers to the death of the body cells. Biological death occurs 4–6 minutes after clinical death and can result in permanent brain damage, as well as damage to other vital organs. If CPR can be started immediately after clinical death occurs, the victim may be revived.

ABCDs OF CPR

Cardiopulmonary resuscitation is as simple as ABCD. In fact, the *ABCDs* serve as guides to lifesaving techniques for persons who have stopped breathing and have no pulse.

♦ *A stands for airway.* To open the victim's airway, use the *head-tilt/chin-lift* method (figure 16-3). Put one hand on the victim's forehead and put the fingertips of the other hand under the bony part of the jaw, near the chin. Tilt the head back without closing the victim's mouth. This action prevents the tongue from falling back and blocking the air passage. If the vic-

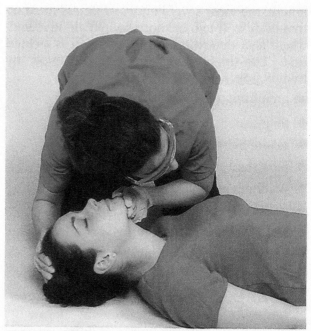

FIGURE 16-3 Open the airway by using the head-tilt/chin-lift method.

tim has a suspected neck or upper spinal cord injury, try to open the airway by lifting the chin without tilting the head back. If it is difficult to keep the jaw lifted with one hand, use a *jaw-thrust maneuver* to open the airway. Assume a position at the victim's head and rest your elbows on the surface on which the victim is lying. Grasp the angles of the victim's lower jaw by positioning one hand on each side. Lift with both hands to move the lower jaw forward, making every attempt to avoid excessive backward tilting or side-to-side movement of the head.

♦ *B stands for breathing.* Breathing means that you breathe into the victim's mouth or nose to supply needed oxygen or provide ventilations. To avoid loss of air when providing mouth-to-mouth breathing, it is important to pinch the victim's nose shut and make a tight seal around the victim's mouth with your mouth. Each breath should take about 1 second and the chest should rise. Rapid or forceful breaths should be avoided because they can force air into the esophagus and stomach, causing gastric distension. This can cause serious complications such as vomiting, aspiration of fluids into the lungs, and even pneumonia.

CAUTION: Follow standard precautions. If possible, use a CPR pocket face mask with a one-way valve to provide a barrier and prevent the transmission of disease (figure 16-4). Special training is required for the use of this mask. Other protective barrier face shields are also available.

♦ *C stands for circulation.* By applying pressure to a certain area of the sternum (breastbone), the heart is compressed between the sternum and vertebral column. Blood is squeezed out of the heart and into the blood vessels. In this way, oxygen is supplied to body cells.

♦ *D stands for defibrillation.* One of the most common causes of cardiac arrest is ventricular fibrillation, an arrhythmia, or abnormal electrical conduction pattern in the heart. When the heart is fibrillating, it does not pump blood effectively. A defibrillator is a machine that delivers an electric shock to the heart to try to restore the normal electrical pattern and rhythm. Automated external defibrillators (AEDs) are now available for use by trained first responders, emergency medical technicians, and even citizens (figure 16-5). After electrode pads are positioned on the victim's chest, the AED determines the heart rhythm, recognizes abnormal rhythms that may respond to defibrillation, and sounds an audible or visual warning telling the operator to push a "shock" button. Some AEDs are fully automatic and even administer the shock. Anytime a shock is administered with an AED, it is essential to make sure no one is touching the victim. The rescuer should state "Clear the victim," and look carefully to make sure no one is in contact with the victim before pushing the shock button. Serious injuries, such as cardiac arrest, could occur in other rescuers if they are shocked by the AED. Newer models of

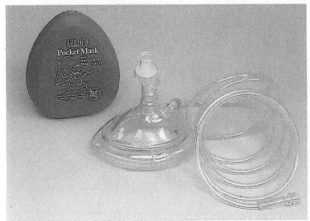

FIGURE 16-4 Whenever possible, use a CPR barrier mask to prevent transmission of disease while giving respirations. The tubing on the mask can be connected to an oxygen supply.

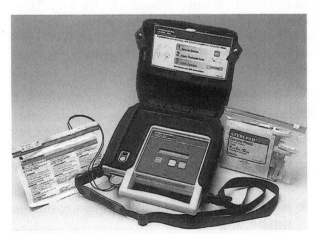

FIGURE 16-5 When cardiac arrest occurs, an automated external defibrillator (AED) can be used to analyze the electrical rhythm of the heart and to apply a shock to try to restore the normal heart rhythm.

AEDs allow the rescuer to deliver either adult or child defibrillator shocks. By using smaller pediatric electrodes and/or a switch on the AED, the rescuer can deliver a smaller electrical shock. The pediatric dose is recommended for any child from 1–8 years of age. The adult defibrillator dose and adult electrodes should be used for any child 8 years or older. In addition, if an AED does not have the option of a pediatric dosage, the adult dosage and electrodes should be used on the child. Currently, there is no recommendation for or against the use of AEDs in infants younger than 1 year. Studies have shown that the sooner defibrillation is provided, the greater the chances of survival are from a cardiac arrest caused by an arrhythmia. However, it is essential to remember that CPR is used until an AED is available. CPR will circulate the blood and prevent biological death.

It is important to know and follow the ABCDs in proper sequence while administering CPR.

BASIC PRINCIPLES OF CPR

Extreme care must be taken to evaluate the victim's condition before CPR is started. The first step is to determine whether the victim is conscious. Tap the victim gently and ask, "Are you OK?" If you know the victim, call the victim by name and speak loudly. If there is no response and the victim is unconscious, call for help. The American Heart Association and the American Red Cross recommend a *"call first, call fast"* priority. If you are alone, *call first* before providing any care to:

◆ an unconscious adult

◆ an unconscious child who has reached puberty as defined by the presence of secondary sex characteristics

◆ an unconscious infant or child with a high risk for heart problems

◆ any victim for whom you witness a sudden cardiac arrest

If you are alone, shout for help, and start CPR if needed for:

◆ an unconscious infant or child from 1 year of age to puberty

◆ any victim of submersion or near drowning

◆ any victim with cardiac arrest caused by a drug overdose or trauma

If no help arrives to call EMS, administer five cycles of CPR (about 2 minutes), and then *call fast* for EMS. Return to the victim immediately to continue providing care until EMS arrives.

After determining that a victim is unconscious, the second step is to check for breathing. Try not to move the victim while you check breathing. If the victim is breathing, leave the victim in the same position and proceed with other needed care. If the victim is not breathing, or you are unable to determine whether the victim is breathing, position the victim on his or her back. If you must turn the victim, support the victim's head and neck, and keep the victim's body in as straight a line as possible while turning (figure 16-6). Then, open the airway by using the head-tilt/chin-lift or, if a neck or spinal cord injury is suspected, the jaw-thrust maneuver. This step will sometimes start the victim breathing. To check for breathing, use a three-point evaluation for at least 5 but not more than 10 seconds. *Look* for chest movement. *Listen* for breathing through the nose or mouth. *Feel* for movement of air from the nose or mouth. If the victim is not breathing, give two breaths, each breath lasting approximately 1 second. Make sure the breaths are effective by watching for the victim's chest to rise. Do *not* give breaths too quickly or with too much

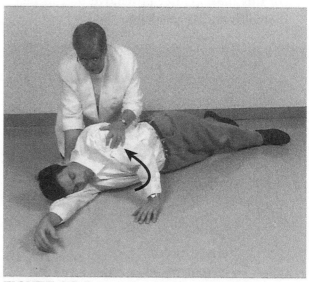

FIGURE 16-6 To turn a victim, support the victim's head and neck, and keep the victim's body in as straight a line as possible.

force because this can cause gastric distension. Pause very briefly between breaths to allow air flow back out of the lungs. In addition, take a breath between the two breaths to increase the oxygen content of the rescue breath.

After giving two breaths, check the carotid pulse in the neck to determine whether cardiac compression is needed. Take at least 5 but no more than 10 seconds to determine whether the pulse is absent before starting compressions.

▽ **CAUTION:** Cardiac compressions are not given if the pulse can be felt. If a person has stopped breathing but still has a pulse, it may be necessary to give only pulmonary respiration.

Correct hand placement is essential before performing chest compressions. For adults, the hand is placed on the lower half of the sternum between the nipples. While kneeling alongside the victim, find the correct position by using the middle finger of your hand that is closest to the victim's feet to follow the ribs up to where the ribs meet the sternum, at the substernal notch (figure 16-7A). Keep the middle finger on the notch and position the index finger above it so two fingers are on the sternum. Then place the heel of your opposite hand (the hand closest to the victim's head) on the sternum, next to the index finger (figure 16-7B). Measuring in this manner minimizes the danger of applying pressure to the tip of the sternum, called the *xiphoid process.*

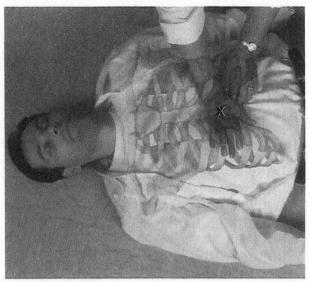

FIGURE 16-7B Place the heel of your opposite hand two fingers' width above the substernal notch. This should place the hand on the lower half of the sternum between the nipples.

▽ **CAUTION:** The xiphoid process can be broken off quite easily and therefore should not be pressed.

After positioning your hands on the sternum, straighten your arms and align your shoulders directly over your hands. To give compressions, push straight down on the victim's sternum with a hard, fast motion. On an adult, the sternum should be compressed 1½ to 2 inches. After each compression, allow the chest to recoil completely. Deliver compressions at a rate of 100 compressions per minute. Proper administration of compressions will produce adequate blood flow and improve the victim's chances of survival.

CPR FOR ADULTS, INFANTS, AND CHILDREN

Cardiopulmonary resuscitation can be performed on adults, children, and infants. In addition, it can be done by one person or two persons. Rates of ventilations and compressions vary according to the number of persons giving CPR and the age of the victim.

◆ *One-person adult rescue:* For adults, a lone rescuer should provide 30 compressions followed by 2 ventilations, for a cycle ratio of 30:2. Compressions should be hard, fast, and

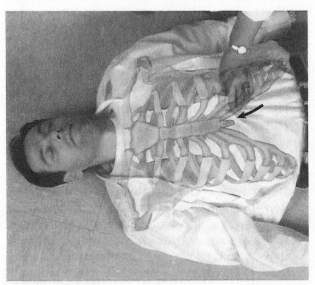

FIGURE 16-7A To position hands correctly for chest compressions, first use a finger to follow the ribs up to where they meet the sternum at the substernal notch.

deep, and given at the rate of approximately 100 per minute. Five 30:2 cycles should be completed every 2 minutes. The hands should be positioned correctly on the sternum. The two hands should be interlaced and only the heel of the palm should rest on the sternum. Pressure should be applied straight down to compress the sternum approximately 1½ to 2 inches, or 3.8 to 5.0 centimeters.

◆ *Two-person adult rescue*: Two people performing a rescue on an adult victim allows one person to give breaths while the second person provides compressions. During the rescue, the person giving breaths can check the effectiveness of the compressions by feeling for a carotid pulse while chest compressions are administered. One rescuer applies the compressions at the rate of 100 per minute. After every 30 compressions, the second rescuer provides 2 ventilations. Thus, there is a 30:2 ratio.

◆ *Infants*: Cardiopulmonary resuscitation for an infant is given to any infant from birth to 1 year of age. It is different than that for an adult because of the infant's size. To open the airway, use a head-tilt/chin-lift method, but the infant's head should not be tilted as far back as an adult's because this can obstruct the infant's airway. Ventilations are given by covering both the infant's nose and mouth; a seal is made by the mouth of the rescuer. Breaths are given until the infant's chest visibly rises. Extreme care must be taken to avoid overinflating the lungs and/or forcing air into the stomach. The brachial pulse site in the arm is used to check pulse (figure 16-8). Compressions are given by placing two fingers on the lower half of the sternum just below an imaginary line drawn between the nipples. The sternum should be compressed about ⅓ to ½ of the depth of the chest. Compressions are given at a rate of 100 per minute. A lone rescuer gives 30 compressions followed by 2 respirations for a 30:2 ratio. The infant's back must be supported at all times when giving compressions. If two rescuers are available to perform CPR on an infant, a two-thumb technique can be used by one rescuer to perform compressions while the second rescuer gives breaths. The rescuer providing compressions

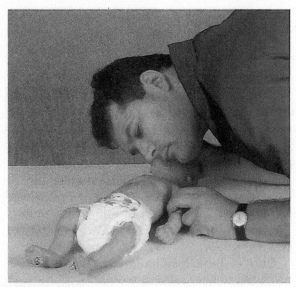

FIGURE 16-8 Use the brachial pulse site in the arm to check for a pulse in an infant.

stands at the infant's feet and places his or her thumbs next to each other on the lower half of the sternum just below the nipple line. The rescuer then wraps his or her hands around the infant to support the infant's back with the fingers. A ratio of 15 compressions to 2 ventilations is used by the two rescuers.

◆ *Children*: Cardiopulmonary resuscitation for children depends on the size of the child. Health care providers should use child CPR methods for any child from 1 year of age to puberty. If a child shows signs of puberty, as evidenced by secondary sex characteristics, adult CPR methods should be used. The initial steps of CPR for a child are the same steps used in adult CPR, except that the head is not tilted as far back when the airway is opened. The main differences relate to compressions. The heel of one hand (or two hands) is placed on the lower half of the sternum in the same position used for adult compressions. If only one hand is used, the other hand remains on the forehead to keep the airway open. The sternum is compressed ⅓ to ½ the depth of the chest. Compressions are given at a rate of 100 per minute. After each set of 30 compressions, 2 breaths are given until the chest visibly rises. This provides a 30:2 ratio. Approximately five cycles of CPR should be completed every 2 minutes.

CHOKING VICTIMS

A choking victim has an obstructed airway (an object blocking the airway). Special measures must be taken to clear this obstruction.

♦ If the victim is conscious, coughing, talking or making noise, and/or able to breathe, the airway is not completely obstructed. Remain calm and encourage the victim to remain calm. Encourage the victim to cough hard. Coughing is the most effective method of expelling the object from the airway.

♦ If the victim is conscious but not able to talk, make noise, breathe, or cough, the airway is completely obstructed. The victim usually grasps his or her throat and appears cyanotic (blue discoloration of the skin) (figure 16-9). Immediate action must be taken to clear the airway. Abdominal thrusts, as described in Procedure 16:2E, are given to provide a force of air to push the object out of the airway.

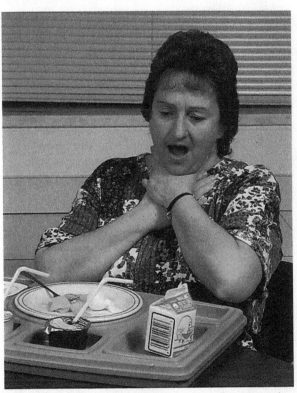

FIGURE 16-9 A choking victim usually grasps her throat and appears cyanotic.

♦ If the victim is unconscious and has an obstructed airway, administer adult CPR. The only change to the adult CPR method is that every time the airway is opened to give breaths, the rescuer should look in the victim's mouth for the object. If the object is visible, the rescuer should use a C-shaped or hooking motion to remove the object. If the object is not seen, the rescuer should try to administer breaths and then continue with chest compressions.

♦ If an infant (birth to 1 year old) has an obstructed airway, a different sequence of steps is used to remove the obstruction. The sequence includes five back blows; five chest thrusts; a check of the mouth; a finger sweep, if the object is seen; and an attempt to ventilate. The sequence, described in detail in Procedure 16:2F, is repeated until the object is expelled, ventilations are successful, or other qualified medical help arrives.

♦ If a child aged 1 to puberty has an obstructed airway, the same sequence of steps used for an adult is followed. A finger sweep of the mouth is *not* performed unless the object can be seen in the mouth.

Once CPR is started, it must be continued unless one of the following situations occur:

♦ The victim recovers and starts to breathe.

♦ Other qualified help arrives and takes over.

♦ A doctor or other legally qualified person orders you to discontinue the attempt.

♦ The rescuer is so physically exhausted, CPR can no longer be continued.

♦ The scene suddenly becomes unsafe.

♦ You are given a legally valid do not resuscitate (DNR) order.

STUDENT: *Go to the workbook and complete the assignment sheet for 16:2, Performing Cardiopulmonary Resuscitation. Then return and continue with the procedures.*

PROCEDURE 16:2A

Performing CPR—One-Person Adult Rescue

Equipment and Supplies

CPR manikin, alcohol or disinfecting solution, gauze sponges

Procedure

⚠ **CAUTION:** Only a CPR training manikin (figure 16-10) should be used to practice this procedure. *Never* practice CPR on another person.

1. Assemble equipment. Position the manikin on a firm surface, usually the floor.

2. *Check for consciousness.* Shake the "victim" by tapping the shoulder. Ask, "Are you OK?" If the victim does not respond, activate EMS immediately. Follow the "call first, call fast" priority. Get an AED if available.

3. *Open the airway.* Use the head-tilt/chin-lift method. Place one hand on the victim's forehead. Place the fingertips of the other hand under the bony part of the victim's jaw, near the chin. Tilt the head without closing the victim's mouth.

NOTE: This action moves the tongue away from the back of the throat and prevents the tongue from blocking the airway.

⚠ **CAUTION:** If the victim has a suspected neck or upper spinal cord injury, use a jaw-thrust maneuver to open the airway. Assume a position on either side of the patient's head. Grasp the angles of the victim's lower jaw by positioning one hand on each side. Lift with both hands to move the lower jaw forward, making every attempt to avoid excessive backward tilting or side-to-side movement of the head.

4. *Check for breathing.* Put your ear close to the victim's nose and mouth while looking at the chest. Look, listen, and feel for respirations for at least 5 but not more than 10 seconds (figure 16-11A).

5. *If the victim is breathing,* keep the airway open and obtain medical help. *If the victim is not breathing,* administer mouth-to-mouth resuscitation as follows:

   a. Keep the airway open.

   b. Resting your hand on the victim's forehead, use your thumb and forefinger to pinch the victim's nose shut.

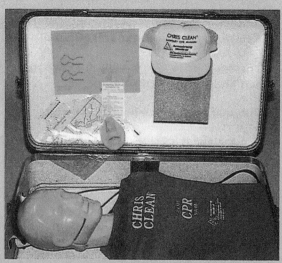

FIGURE 16-10 Use only training manikins while practicing CPR.

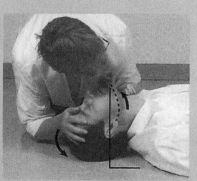

FIGURE 16-11A Open the airway and take at least 5 but no more than 10 seconds to look, listen, and feel for breathing.

PROCEDURE 16:2A

c. Seal the victim's mouth with your mouth or position your mouth on the barrier mask.

d. Give two breaths, each lasting approximately 1 second until the chest visibly rises (figure 16-11B). Pause slightly between breaths. This allows air to flow out and provides you with a chance to take a breath and increase the oxygen level for the second rescue breath.

e. Watch the chest for movement to be sure the air is entering the victim's lungs. Avoid overinflating the lungs and/or forcing air into the stomach.

CAUTION: Follow standard precautions. If possible, use a CPR pocket face mask with a one-way valve to provide a barrier and prevent the transmission of disease.

CAUTION: Giving breaths too quickly or with too much force can cause gastric distention. This can lead to serious complications such as vomiting, aspiration of fluids into the lungs, and pneumonia.

6. *Palpate the carotid pulse.* Kneeling at the victim's side, place the fingertips of your hand on the victim's voice box. Then slide the fingers toward you and into the groove at the side of the victim's neck, where you should find the carotid pulse. Take at least 5 seconds but not

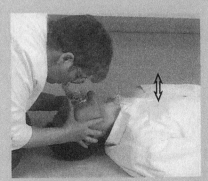

FIGURE 16-11B If the victim is not breathing, open the airway and give two breaths. Watch for the chest to visibly rise.

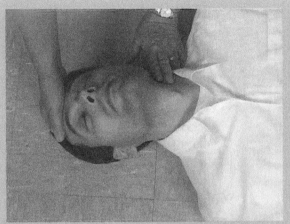

FIGURE 16-11C Palpate the carotid pulse for at least 5 but not more than 10 seconds to determine whether the heart is beating.

more than 10 seconds to feel for the pulse (figure 16-11C). At the same time, watch for breathing, signs of circulation, and/or movement.

NOTE: The pulse may be weak, so check carefully.

7. *If the victim has a pulse, continue providing mouth-to-mouth resuscitation.* Give one breath every 5–6 seconds. Count, "One, one thousand; two, one thousand; three, one thousand; four, one thousand; and breathe," to obtain the correct timing. Recheck the pulse every 2 minutes to make sure the heart is still beating.

8. *If the victim does not have a pulse, administer chest compressions* as follows:

a. Locate the correct place on the sternum. While kneeling alongside the victim, use the middle finger of your hand that is closest to the victim's feet to follow the ribs up to where the ribs meet the sternum, at the substernal notch. Keep the middle finger on the notch and position the index finger above it so two fingers are on the sternum. Then, place the heel of the opposite hand (the one closest to the victim's head) on the sternum, next to the index finger.

PROCEDURE 16:2A

 CAUTION: The heel of your hand should be on the lower half of the sternum at the nipple line.

b. Place your other hand on top of the hand that is correctly positioned. Keep your fingers off the victim's chest. It may help to interlock your fingers.

c. Rise up on your knees so that your shoulders are directly over the victim's sternum. Lock your elbows and keep your arms straight.

NOTE: This position will allow you to push straight down on the sternum and compress the heart, which lies between the sternum and vertebral column.

d. Push down hard and fast to compress the chest approximately 1½ to 2 inches, or 3.8 to 5.0 centimeters (figure 16-11D). Use a smooth, even motion.

e. Administer 30 compressions at the rate of 100 per minute. Count, "One, two, three," and so forth, to obtain the correct rate.

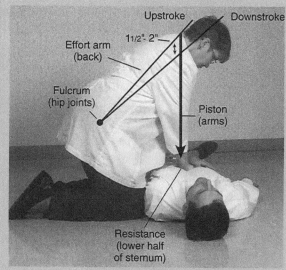

FIGURE 16-11D Use hard and fast motions to compress the chest straight down while giving 30 compressions.

f. Allow the chest to recoil or re-expand completely after each compression. Keep your hands on the sternum during the upstroke (chest relaxation period).

NOTE: When the chest recoils or re-expands completely, this allows more blood to refill the heart between compressions.

9. After administering 30 compressions, give the victim 2 ventilations, or respirations. Avoid excessive body movement while giving the ventilations. Keep your knees in the same position and swing your body upward to give the respirations.

NOTE: Make every effort to minimize any interruptions to chest compressions. There is no blood flow to the brain and heart when compressions are not being performed.

10. Continue the cycles of 30 compressions followed by 2 ventilations until EMS providers take over, an AED arrives, or the victim recovers.

11. If an automated external defibrillator (AED) is available, give five cycles of CPR and then use the AED. Even though AEDs have different manufacturers and models, they all operate in basically the same way.

a. Position the AED at the victim's side next to the rescuer who is using it. If another person arrives to help, the second person can activate EMS (if this has not already been done) and then administer cycles of CPR on the victim's other side.

b. Open the case on the AED and turn on the power control.

NOTE: Some AEDs power on automatically when the case is opened.

c. Expose the victim's chest and attach the chest electrodes to bare skin. If

PROCEDURE 16:2A

the chest is covered with sweat or water, quickly wipe it dry. Choose the correct size electrode pad. Use adult size pads for any victim 8 years and older. Peel the backing off of the electrode pad. Place one pad on the upper right side of the chest, below the clavicle (collarbone) and to the right of the sternum (breastbone). Place the second electrode pad on the left side of the chest to the left of the nipple and a few inches below the axillae (armpit).

d. If necessary, attach the connecting cables of the electrodes to the electrode pad and AED. Some types of electrodes are preconnected.

e. Clearly state "Clear the victim." Look carefully to make sure no one is touching the victim. Push the analyze control to allow the AED to evaluate the heart rhythm (figure 16–12). The analysis may take 5–15 seconds.

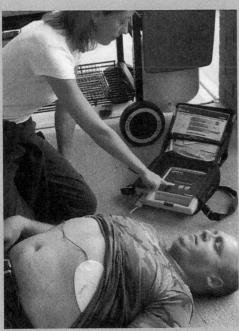

FIGURE 16-12 "Clear" the victim before pushing the control to allow the automated external defibrillator (AED) to analyze the victim's heart rhythm.

f. Follow the recommendations of the AED. If the AED says NO SHOCK, resume CPR by giving 30 compressions followed by 2 ventilations.

g. If the AED says SHOCK, make sure the victim is clear. Loudly state "Clear victim," and look to make sure no one is touching the victim. Push the shock button.

CAUTION: If another rescuer is touching the victim, the rescuer will also receive the shock. This can cause a serious injury and/or a cardiac arrest.

h. Begin cycles of CPR by starting with chest compressions immediately after the shock is delivered to the victim. After 2 minutes of CPR, most AEDs will prompt you to reanalyze the rhythm and deliver additional shocks if necessary.

12. After you begin CPR, do not stop unless

a. the victim recovers

b. help arrives to take over and give CPR and/or apply an AED

c. a physician or other legally qualified person orders you to discontinue the attempt

d. you are so physically exhausted, you cannot continue

e. the scene suddenly becomes unsafe

f. you are given a legally valid do not resuscitate (DNR) order

13. After the practice session, use a gauze pad saturated with 70-percent alcohol or a 10-percent bleach disinfecting solution to clean the manikin. Wipe the face and clean inside the mouth thoroughly. Saturate a clean gauze pad with the solution and lay it on the mouth area for at least 30 seconds. Use another gauze pad to wipe the area dry. Follow manufacturer's instructions for any additional cleaning required.

PROCEDURE 16:2A

NOTE: A 10-percent bleach solution is more effective than alcohol. Some manikins have disposable mouthpieces that are discarded after use. If the mouthpiece is discarded, the remainder of the face should still be disinfected.

14. Replace all equipment used. Wash hands.

✓ **Final Checkpoint** Using the criteria listed on the evaluation sheet, your instructor will grade your performance.

Practice

Go to the workbook and use the evaluation sheet for 16:2A, Performing CPR—One-Person Adult Rescue, to practice this procedure. When you believe you have mastered this skill, sign the sheet and give it to your instructor for further action.

PROCEDURE 16:2B

Performing CPR— Two-Person Adult Rescue

Equipment and Supplies

CPR manikin, alcohol or disinfecting solution, gauze sponges

Procedure

▽ **CAUTION:** Only a CPR training manikin should be used to practice this procedure. *Never* practice CPR on another person.

1. Assemble equipment. Position the manikin on a firm surface, usually the floor.

2. Shake the victim to check for consciousness. Ask, "Are you OK?"

3. If the victim is unconscious, one rescuer checks for breathing and begins CPR. The second rescuer activates emergency medical services and obtains an AED if available.

4. Use the head-tilt/chin-lift method to open the victim's airway. Place one hand on the victim's forehead. Place the fingertips of the other hand under the bony part of the victim's jaw, near the chin. Tilt the victim's head back without closing the victim's mouth.

5. Check for breathing. Look, listen, and feel for breathing for at least 5 but not more than 10 seconds.

6. *If the victim is not breathing,* give two breaths, each lasting approximately 1 second. Watch the chest for movement to be sure air is entering the victim's lungs. Avoid overinflating the lungs and/or forcing air into the stomach.

⊞ **CAUTION:** Follow standard precautions. If possible, use a CPR pocket face mask with a one-way valve to provide a barrier and prevent the transmission of disease.

7. Feel for the carotid pulse for at least 5 seconds and not more than 10 seconds. Watch for signs of breathing, circulation, and/or movement.

8. *If there is no pulse,* give chest compressions. Locate the correct hand position on the sternum. Until the second rescuer returns, provide compressions and respirations as for a one-person rescue. Give 30 hard, fast, and deep compressions followed by 2 respirations.

PROCEDURE 16:2B

9. When the second rescuer returns after calling for help, the first rescuer should complete the cycle of 30 compressions and 2 respirations.

10. The second rescuer should get into position for compressions and locate the correct hand placement while the first rescuer is giving the two breaths. The second rescuer should begin compressions at the rate of 100 per minute (figure 16-13A). The second rescuer should count out loud, "One, two, three, four, five . . ." After each set of 30 compressions, the second rescuer should pause very briefly to allow the first rescuer to give 2 breaths. Rescue then continues with 2 breaths after each 30 compressions.

11. After every five cycles of CPR (approximately 2 minutes) the rescuers should change positions. The person giving compressions can provide a clear signal to change positions, such as, "Change, two, three, four. . . ." The compressor should complete a cycle of 30 compressions. The ventilator should give 2 breaths at the end of the 30 compressions. The ventilator should then move to the chest and locate the correct hand placement

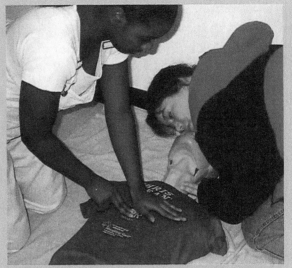

FIGURE 16-13B Rescuers should change positions after every five cycles of CPR because the person doing compressions gets tired, and compressions are not as effective.

for compressions (figure 16-13B). The compressor should move to the head and open the airway. The new compressor should then give 30 hard, fast, and deep compressions at the rate of 100 per minute. The rescue should continue with 2 ventilations after each 30 compressions.

12. If an AED is available, one rescuer should set up the AED while the other rescuer is giving cycles of CPR. When the AED is ready to analyze the heart rhythm, the rescuer operating the AED must make sure the other rescuer is clear of the victim. The steps for using the AED are discussed in detail in step 11 of Procedure 16:2A.

13. The rescuers should continue CPR until qualified medical help arrives, the victim recovers, a doctor or other legally qualified person orders CPR discontinued, the scene suddenly becomes unsafe, or they are presented with a legally valid do not resuscitate (DNR) order.

14. After the practice session, use a gauze pad saturated with 70-percent alcohol

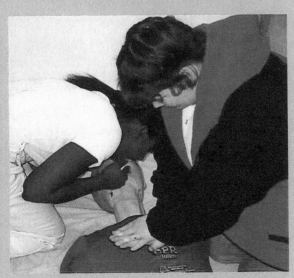

FIGURE 16-13A In a two-person rescue, two breaths are given after every 30 compressions.

PROCEDURE 16:2B

or a 10-percent bleach disinfecting solution to clean the manikin. Wipe the face and clean inside the mouth thoroughly. Saturate a clean gauze pad with the solution and lay it on the mouth area for at least 30 seconds. Use another gauze pad to wipe the area dry. Follow manufacturer's instructions for any additional cleaning required.

NOTE: A 10-percent bleach solution is more effective than alcohol. Some manikins have disposable mouthpieces that are discarded after use. If the mouthpiece is discarded, the remainder of the face should still be disinfected.

15. Replace all equipment used. Wash hands.

Practice

Go to the workbook and use the evaluation sheet for 16:2B, Performing CPR—Two-Person Adult Rescue, to practice this procedure. When you believe you have mastered this skill, sign the sheet and give it to your instructor for further action.

 Final Checkpoint Using the criteria listed on the evaluation sheet, your instructor will grade your performance.

PROCEDURE 16:2C

Performing CPR on Infants

Equipment and Supplies

CPR infant manikin, alcohol or disinfecting solution, gauze pads

Procedure

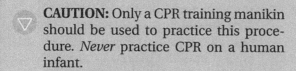 **CAUTION:** Only a CPR training manikin should be used to practice this procedure. *Never* practice CPR on a human infant.

1. Assemble equipment.

2. Gently shake the infant or tap the infant's foot (for reflex action) to determine consciousness. Call to the infant.

   NOTE: For CPR techniques, infants are usually considered to be under 1 year old.

3. If the infant is unconscious, call aloud for help, and begin the steps of CPR. If no one arrives to call EMS, stop CPR after five cycles (approximately 2 minutes) to telephone for medical assistance. Resume CPR as quickly as possible.

   NOTE: If the infant is known to have a high risk for heart problems or a sudden collapse was witnessed, activate EMS and then begin CPR.

4. Use the head-tilt/chin-lift method to open the infant's airway. Tip the head back gently, taking care not to tip it as far back as you would an adult's head.

   CAUTION: Tipping the head too far will cause an obstruction of the infant's airway.

5. Look, listen, and feel for breathing (figure 16-14A). Check for at least 5 but not more than 10 seconds.

6. *If there is no breathing,* give two breaths, each breath lasting approximately 1 second. Cover the infant's nose and mouth with your mouth. Breathe until the chest

PROCEDURE 16:2C

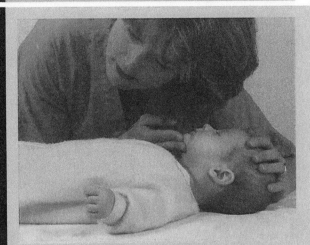

FIGURE 16-14A Look, listen, and feel for breathing for at least 5 but not more than 10 seconds.

rises visibly during each ventilation. Allow for chest deflation after each breath.

7. Check the pulse over the brachial artery. Place your fingertips on the inside of the upper arm and halfway between the elbow and shoulder (figure 16-14B). Put your thumb on the posterior (outside) of the arm. Squeeze your fingers gently toward your thumb. Feel for the pulse for at least 5 but not more than 10 seconds.

8. *If a pulse is present,* continue providing ventilations by giving the infant one ventilation every 3 seconds (approximately 20 breaths per minute). Recheck the pulse every 2 minutes.

9. *If no pulse is present or if the heart rate is below 60 beats per minute with signs of poor circulation such as cyanosis,* administer cardiac compressions. Locate the correct position for compressions by drawing an imaginary line between the nipples. Place two fingers on the sternum just below this imaginary line. Give compressions at the rate of 100 per minute (figure 16-14C). Make sure the infant is on a firm surface, or use one hand to support the infant's back while administering compressions. Press hard, fast, and deep enough to compress the infant's chest ⅓ to ½ the depth of the chest. Give 30 compressions at the rate of 100 per minute. Allow the chest to recoil or re-expand completely between compressions.

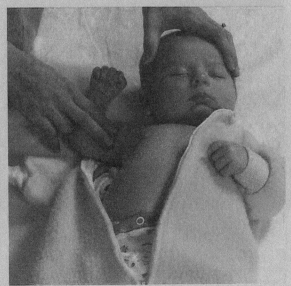

FIGURE 16-14B Check the pulse at the brachial artery in the upper arm.

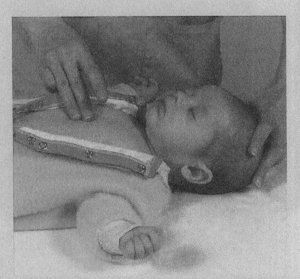

FIGURE 16-14C Use two fingers to give hard and fast compressions to the infant, at a rate of 100 compressions per minute.

PROCEDURE 16:2C

10. After every 30 compressions, give 2 breaths until the chest rises visibly.

11. Continue the cycle of 30 compressions followed by 2 ventilations. To establish the correct rate, count, "One, two, three, four, five."

12. If a second rescuer arrives to assist, the second rescuer should activate EMS if this has not been done. Then both rescuers can perform CPR on the infant.

    a. The first rescuer should finish a cycle of 30 compressions followed by 2 respirations.

    b. The second rescuer should stand at the infant's feet and place his or her thumbs next to each other on the lower half of the sternum just below the nipple line. The rescuer then wraps his or her hands around the infant to support the infant's back with the fingers, and uses the thumbs to administer 15 compressions.

    c. After 15 compressions, the person giving compressions pauses very briefly so the other rescuer can give 2 ventilations.

    NOTE: The ratio of compressions to ventilations is 15:2 for a two-person rescue on an infant.

    d. The rescuers should switch positions after every six to eight cycles (approximately 2 minutes) of CPR.

13. The rescuers should continue the cycles of CPR until qualified medical help arrives, the infant recovers, a doctor or other legally qualified person orders CPR discontinued, or they are presented with a legally valid do not resuscitate (DNR) order (very rare for infants).

14. After the practice session, use a gauze pad saturated with 70-percent alcohol or a 10-percent bleach disinfecting solution to clean the manikin. Wipe the face and clean inside the mouth thoroughly. Saturate a clean gauze pad with the solution and lay it on the mouth area for at least 30 seconds. Use another gauze pad to wipe the area dry. Follow manufacturer's instructions for specific cleaning.

    NOTE: The 10-percent bleach solution is more effective than alcohol. Some manikins have disposable mouthpieces that are discarded after use. If the mouthpiece is discarded, the remainder of the face should still be disinfected.

15. Replace all equipment used. Wash hands.

Practice

Go to the workbook and use the evaluation sheet for 16:2C, Performing CPR on Infants to practice this procedure. When you believe you have mastered this skill, sign the sheet and give it to your instructor for further action.

✔ **Final Checkpoint** Using the criteria listed on the evaluation sheet, your instructor will grade your performance.

PROCEDURE 16:2D

Performing CPR on Children

Equipment and Supplies

CPR child manikin, alcohol or disinfecting solution, gauze pads

Procedure

▽ **CAUTION:** Only a CPR training manikin should be used to practice this procedure. *Never* practice CPR on a human child.

1. Assemble equipment.

2. Gently shake the child to determine consciousness. Call to the child.

   NOTE: Health care providers should use child CPR techniques on any child from 1 year of age to puberty, as evidenced by the development of secondary sex characteristics.

3. If the child is unconscious, call aloud for help, and begin the steps of CPR. If no one arrives to call EMS, stop CPR after five cycles (approximately 2 minutes) to telephone for medical assistance and obtain an AED if available. Resume CPR as quickly as possible.

   NOTE: If the child is known to have a high risk for heart problems or a sudden collapse was witnessed, activate EMS first and then begin CPR.

4. Use the head-tilt/chin-lift method to open the child's airway. Tip the head back gently, taking care not to tip it as far back as you would an adult's head.

5. Look, listen, and feel for breathing. Check for at least 5 but not more than 10 seconds.

6. *If there is no breathing,* give two breaths, each breath lasting approximately 1 second. Cover the child's nose and mouth with your mouth, or pinch the child's nose and cover the child's mouth with your mouth. Breathe until the chest rises visibly during each ventilation. Allow for chest deflation after each breath.

7. Check the pulse at the carotid pulse site. Feel for the pulse for at least 5 but not more than 10 seconds.

8. *If a pulse is present,* continue providing ventilations by giving the child one ventilation every 3 seconds (approximately 20 breaths per minute). Recheck the pulse every 2 minutes.

9. *If no pulse is present or if the heart rate is below 60 beats per minute with signs of poor circulation such as cyanosis,* administer cardiac compressions. Place the heel of one hand on the lower half of the sternum just below a line drawn between the nipples or in the same position used for adult CPR. Keep the other hand on the child's forehead (figure 16-15). If the child is larger, two hands can be posi-

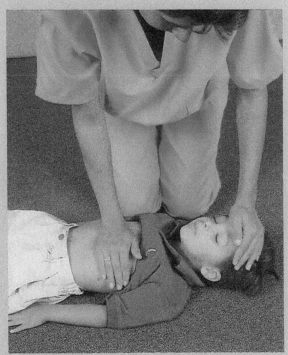

FIGURE 16-15 Use one hand to give chest compressions to a child. Keep the other hand on the child's forehead.

PROCEDURE 16:2D

tioned on the chest for compressions. Give compressions at the rate of 100 per minute. Make sure the child is on a firm surface, or use one hand to support the child's back while administering compressions. Press hard, fast, and deep enough to compress the child's chest ⅓ to ½ the depth of the chest. Give 30 compressions at the rate of 100 per minute. Allow the chest to recoil or re-expand completely between compressions.

10. After every 30 compressions, give 2 breaths until the chest rises visibly.

11. Continue the cycle of 30 compressions followed by 2 ventilations. To establish the correct rate, count, "One, two, three, four, five."

12. If a second rescuer arrives to assist, the second rescuer should activate EMS if this has not been done. Then both rescuers can perform CPR on the child.

    a. The first rescuer should finish a cycle of 30 compressions followed by 2 respirations.

    b. The second rescuer should locate the proper position on the sternum for compressions. As soon as the first rescuer delivers the 2 respirations, the second rescuer should administer 15 compressions.

    c. After 15 compressions, the person giving compressions pauses very briefly so the other rescuer can give 2 ventilations.

    NOTE: The ratio of compressions to ventilations is 15:2 for a two-person rescue on a child.

    d. The rescuers should switch positions after every six to eight cycles (approximately 2 minutes) of CPR.

13. If an AED is available, one rescuer should set up the AED while the other rescuer is giving cycles of CPR. When the AED is ready to analyze the heart rhythm, the rescuer operating the AED must make sure the other rescuer is clear of the vic-

tim. The steps for using the AED are discussed in detail in step 11 of Procedure 16:2A.

⚠ **CAUTION:** Adult electrode pads should be used on any child 8 years or older. Child or pediatric electrodes are used only on children from 1–8 years of age.

14. The rescuers should continue the cycles of CPR until qualified medical help arrives, the child recovers, a doctor or other legally qualified person orders CPR discontinued, or they are presented with a legally valid do not resuscitate (DNR) order.

15. After the practice session, use a gauze pad saturated with 70-percent alcohol or a 10-percent bleach disinfecting solution to clean the manikin. Wipe the face and clean inside the mouth thoroughly. Saturate a clean gauze pad with the solution and lay it on the mouth area for at least 30 seconds. Use another gauze pad to wipe the area dry. Follow manufacturer's instructions for specific cleaning.

    NOTE: The 10-percent bleach solution is more effective than alcohol. Some manikins have disposable mouthpieces that are discarded after use. If the mouthpiece is discarded, the remainder of the face should still be disinfected.

16. Replace all equipment used. Wash hands.

Practice

Go to the workbook and use the evaluation sheet for 16:2D, Performing CPR on Children, to practice this procedure. When you believe you have mastered this skill, sign the sheet and give it to your instructor for further action.

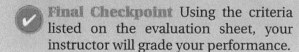 **Final Checkpoint** Using the criteria listed on the evaluation sheet, your instructor will grade your performance.

PROCEDURE 16:2E

Performing CPR— Obstructed Airway on Conscious Adult or Child

Equipment and Supplies

CPR manikin or choking manikin

Procedure

▽ **CAUTION:** Only a manikin should be used to practice this procedure. Do not practice on another person. Hand placement can be tried on another person, but the actual abdominal thrust should *never* be performed unless the person is choking.

1. Assemble equipment. Position the manikin in an upright position sitting on a chair.

2. Determine whether the victim has an airway obstruction. Ask, "Are you choking?" Check to see whether the victim can cough or speak.

▽ **CAUTION:** If the victim is coughing forcefuly, the airway is not completely obstructed. Encourage the victim to remain calm and cough hard. Coughing is usually very effective for removing an obstruction.

3. If the victim cannot cough, talk, make noise, or breathe, call for help.

4. Perform abdominal thrusts to try to remove the obstruction. Follow these steps:

   a. Stand behind the victim.

   b. Wrap both arms around the victim's waist.

   c. Make a fist of one hand (figure 16-16A). Place the thumb side of the fist in the middle of the victim's abdomen, slightly above the navel (umbili-

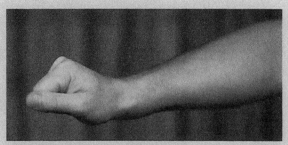

FIGURE 16-16A Make a fist of one hand.

cus) but well below the xiphoid process at the end of the sternum.

   d. Grasp the fist with your other hand (figure 16-16B).

   e. Use quick, upward thrusts to press into the victim's abdomen (figure 16-16C).

NOTE: The thrusts should be delivered hard enough to cause a force of air to push the obstruction out of the airway.

▽ **CAUTION:** Make sure that your forearms do not press against the victim's rib cage while the thrusts are being performed.

   f. If you cannot reach around the victim to give abdominal thrusts (the victim is very obese), or if a victim is in the later stages of pregnancy, give chest thrusts. Stand behind the victim. Wrap your arms under the victim's axilla (armpits) and around to the center of the chest. Make a fist

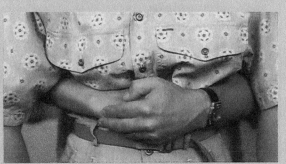

FIGURE 16-16B Place the thumb side of the fist above the umbilicus but well below the xiphoid process at the end of the sternum. Grasp the fist with your other hand.

PROCEDURE 16:2E

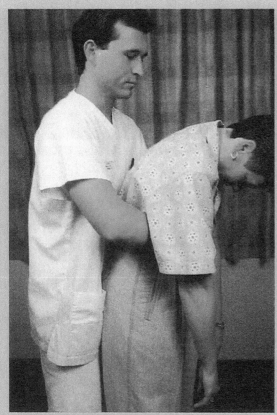

FIGURE 16-16C Use quick, upward thrusts to press into the victim's abdomen.

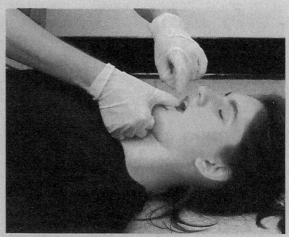

FIGURE 16-17 If an object is visible in the mouth, use a C-shaped, or hooking, motion to remove the object.

with one hand and place the thumb side of the fist against the center of the sternum but well above the xiphoid process. Grab your fist with your other hand and thrust inward.

g. Repeat the thrusts until the object is expelled or until the victim becomes unconscious.

5. If the victim loses consciousness, begin CPR. Activate EMS if this has not already been done. Then start the cycle of CPR by opening the airway and checking breathing. The only difference in CPR for a choking victim is that every time you open the airway you should look in the mouth before giving breaths. If you see an object, use a C-shaped or hooking motion to remove the object (figure 16-17). Perform CPR.

a. Open the airway.

b. Check breathing for at least 5 but not more than 10 seconds.

c. Look in the mouth and remove the object if it is visible.

d. Try giving two breaths.

e. Check the carotid pulse for at least 5 but not more than 10 seconds.

f. If there is a pulse, continue to try to give breaths and check the pulse every 2 minutes.

g. If there is no pulse, give CPR cycles of 30 compressions followed by 2 respirations.

h. Check the mouth for the object every time you are ready to give breaths.

6. Do *not* stop CPR unless the victim recovers, help arrives to take over, a physician or other legally qualified person orders you to discontinue the attempt, you are so physically exhausted you cannot continue, or the scene suddenly becomes unsafe.

7. Make every effort to obtain medical help for the victim as soon as possible.

PROCEDURE 16:2E

8. After the practice session, replace all equipment used. Wash hands.

✓ **Final Checkpoint** Using the criteria listed on the evaluation sheet, your instructor will grade your performance.

Practice

Go to the workbook and use the evaluation sheet for 16:2E, Performing CPR—Obstructed Airway on Conscious Adult or Child, to practice this procedure. When you believe you have mastered this skill, sign the sheet and give it to your instructor for further action.

PROCEDURE 16:2F

Performing CPR— Obstructed Airway on Conscious Infant

Equipment and Supplies

CPR infant manikin, alcohol or disinfecting solution, gauze sponges

Procedure

▽ **CAUTION:** Only an infant manikin should be used to practice this procedure. Do *not* practice on a real infant.

1. Assemble equipment. Kneel or sit with the infant in your lap.

   NOTE: An infant is any baby to 1 year of age. Health care providers should use the adult choking sequence for any child older than 1 year.

2. Shake the infant gently. Ask, "Are you OK?"

3. If the infant is conscious and coughing forcefully, allow the infant to cough. The airway is not completely obstructed and the coughing may expel the object.

4. If the infant cannot cry, make any sounds, is making a high-pitched noise while inhaling or no noise at all, is turning cyanotic, and does not appear to be breathing, the airway is completely obstructed. Activate EMS immediately.

5. Quickly bare the infant's chest to expose the sternum (breastbone).

6. Give five back blows. Hold the infant face down, with your arm supporting the infant's body and your hand supporting the infant's head and jaw. Position the head lower than the chest (figure 16-18A). Use the heel of your other hand to give five firm back blows between the infant's shoulder blades.

▽ **CAUTION:** When performing back blows on an infant, do not use excessive force.

7. Support the infant's head and neck to turn the infant face up. Hold the infant with your forearm resting on your thigh. Keep the infant's head lower than the chest.

8. Give five chest thrusts. Position two to three fingers on the sternum just below

PROCEDURE 16:2F

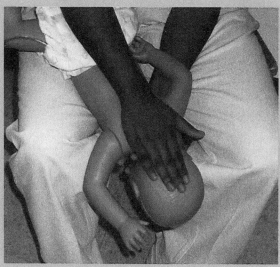

FIGURE 16-18A To give an infant five back blows, position the infant face down, with the head lower than the chest.

an imaginary line drawn between the nipples. Press straight down five times (figure 16-18B), to compress the sternum ⅓ to ½ the depth of the chest.

9. Continue the cycle of five back blows followed by five chest thrusts until EMS arrives or the infant becomes unresponsive.

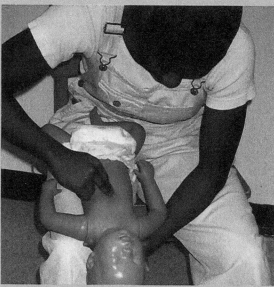

FIGURE 16-18B Give the infant five chest thrusts, keeping the head lower than the chest.

10. If the infant becomes unresponsive, place the infant on a firm surface. Open the airway and look for an object. If an object is visible, use a C-shaped or hooking motion to remove it. Then perform CPR following the normal procedure for an infant, except look in the mouth every time you are ready to give breaths.

    a. Attempt to give two breaths.

    b. Check the brachial pulse for at least 5 but not more than 10 seconds.

    c. If there is a pulse, continue to try to give breaths and check the pulse every 2 minutes.

    d. If there is no pulse, give CPR cycles of 30 compressions followed by 2 respirations.

    e. Check the mouth for the object every time you are ready to give breaths.

11. Do *not* stop CPR unless the infant recovers, help arrives to take over, a physician or other legally qualified person orders you to discontinue the attempt, you are so physically exhausted you cannot continue, or the scene suddenly becomes unsafe.

12. Make every effort to obtain medical help for the infant as soon as possible.

13. After the practice session, use a gauze pad saturated with 70-percent alcohol or a 10-percent bleach disinfecting solution to clean the manikin. Wipe the face and clean inside the mouth thoroughly. Saturate a clean gauze pad with the solution and lay it on the mouth area for at least 30 seconds. Use another gauze pad to wipe the area dry. Follow manufacturer's recommendations for specific cleaning or care.

NOTE: A 10-percent bleach solution is more effective than alcohol. Some manikins have disposable mouthpieces that are discarded after use. If the mouth-

PROCEDURE 16:2F

piece is discarded, the remainder of the face should still be disinfected.

14. Replace all equipment used. Wash hands.

✔ **Final Checkpoint** Using the criteria listed on the evaluation sheet, your instructor will grade your performance.

Practice

Go to the workbook and use the evaluation sheet for 16:2F, Performing CPR—Obstructed Airway on Conscious Infant, to practice this procedure. When you believe you have mastered this skill, sign the sheet and give it to your instructor for further action.

16:3 INFORMATION

Providing First Aid for Bleeding and Wounds

INTRODUCTION

In any health career, as well as in your personal life, you may need to provide first aid to control bleeding or care for wounds. A **wound** involves injury to the soft tissues. Wounds are usually classified as open or closed. With an open wound, there is a break in the skin or mucous membrane. With a closed wound, there is no break in the skin or mucous membrane but injury occurs to the underlying tissues. An example of a closed wound is a bruise or hematoma. Wounds can result in bleeding, infection, and/or tetanus (lockjaw, a serious infection caused by bacteria). First aid care must be directed toward controlling bleeding before the bleeding leads to death, and toward preventing or obtaining treatment for infection.

TYPES OF OPEN WOUNDS

Open wounds are classified into types according to the injuries that occur. Some main types are abrasions, incisions, lacerations, punctures, avulsions, and amputations.

◆ **Abrasion:** With this type of wound the skin is scraped off. Bleeding is usually limited, but infection must be prevented because dirt and contaminants often enter the wound.

◆ **Incision:** This is a cut or injury caused by a sharp object such as a knife, scissors, or razor blade. The edges of the wound are smooth and regular. If the cut is deep, bleeding can be heavy and can lead to excessive blood loss. In addition, damage to muscles, nerves, and other tissues can occur (figure 16-19).

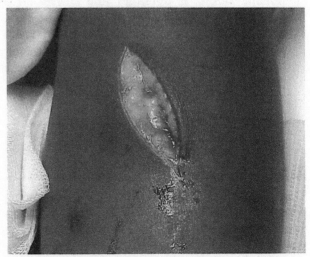

FIGURE 16-19 An incision, caused by a sharp object such as a knife or razor blade, can cause heavy bleeding and/or damage to muscles, nerves, and other tissues. *(Courtesy of Ron Stram, MD, Albany Medical Center, Albany, NY)*

◆ **Laceration:** This type of wound involves tearing of the tissues by way of excessive force. The wound often has jagged, irregular edges. Bleeding may be heavy. If the wound is deep, contamination may lead to infection.

◆ **Puncture:** This type of wound is caused by a sharp object such as a pin, nail, or pointed instrument. Gunshot wounds can also cause puncture wounds that are extremely dangerous because the damage is hidden under the skin and not visible. With all puncture wounds, external bleeding is usually limited, but internal bleeding can occur. In addition, the chance for infection is increased and tetanus may develop if tetanus bacteria enter the wound.

◆ **Avulsion:** This type of wound occurs when tissue is torn or separated from the victim's body. It can result in a piece of torn tissue hanging from the ear, nose, hand, or other body part. Bleeding is heavy and usually extensive. It is important to preserve the body part while caring for this type of wound, because a surgeon may be able to reattach it.

◆ **Amputation:** This type of injury occurs when a body part is cut off and separated from the body. Loss of a finger, toe, hand, or other body part can occur. Bleeding can be heavy and extensive. Care must be taken to preserve the amputated part because a surgeon may be able to reattach it. The part should be wrapped in a cool, moist dressing (use sterile water or normal saline, if possible) and placed in a plastic bag. The plastic bag should be kept cool or placed in ice water and transported with the victim. The body part should never be placed directly on ice because ice can freeze the tissue.

CONTROLLING BLEEDING

Controlling bleeding is the first priority in caring for wounds, because it is possible for a victim to bleed to death in a short period of time. Bleeding can come from arteries, veins, and capillaries. *Arterial blood* usually spurts from a wound, results in heavy blood loss, and is bright red. Arterial bleeding is life-threatening and must be controlled quickly. *Venous blood* is slower, steadier, and dark red or maroon. Venous bleeding is constant and can lead to a large blood loss, but it is easier to control. *Capillary blood* "oozes" from the wound slowly, is less red than arterial blood, and clots easily. The four main methods for controlling bleeding are listed in the order in which they should be used: direct pressure, elevation, pressure bandage, and pressure points.

⊞ **CAUTION:** If possible, use some type of protective barrier, such as gloves or plastic wrap, while controlling bleeding. If this is not possible in an emergency, use thick layers of dressings and try to avoid contact of blood with your skin. Wash your hands thoroughly and as soon as possible after giving first aid to a bleeding victim.

◆ *Direct pressure*: Using your gloved hand over a thick dressing or sterile gauze, apply pressure directly to the wound (figure 16-20A). If no dressing is available, use a clean cloth or linen-type towel. In an emergency when no materials are available, it may even be necessary to use a bare hand. Continue to apply pressure for 5–10 minutes or until the bleeding stops. If blood soaks through the dressing, apply a second dressing over the first and continue to apply direct pressure. Do *not* disturb blood clots once they have formed. Direct pressure will usually stop most bleeding.

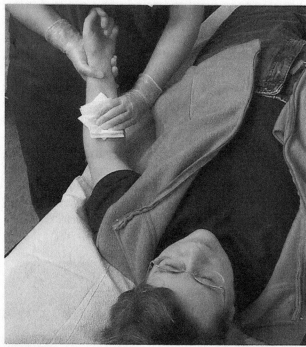

FIGURE 16-20A If possible, use some type of protective barrier, such as gloves or plastic wrap, while applying direct pressure to control bleeding.

◆ *Elevation*: Raise the injured part above the level of the victim's heart to allow gravity to aid in stopping the blood flow from the wound. Continue applying direct pressure while elevating the injured part (figure 16-20B).

🔻 **CAUTION:** If fractures (broken bones) are present or suspected, the part should *not* be elevated.

◆ *Pressure bandage*: Apply a pressure bandage to hold the dressings in place. Maintain direct pressure and elevation while applying the pressure bandage. The procedure for applying a pressure bandage is described in step 4 of Procedure 16:3.

◆ *Pressure points*: If direct pressure, elevation, and the pressure bandage do not stop severe bleeding, it may be necessary to apply pressure to pressure points. By applying pressure to a main artery and pressing it against an underlying bone, the main blood supply to the injured area can be cut off. However, because this technique also stops circulation to other parts of the limb, it should *not* be used any longer than is absolutely necessary. Direct pressure and elevation should also be continued while pressure is being applied to the pressure point.

The main pressure point for the arm is the brachial artery. It is located on the inside of the arm, approximately halfway between the armpit and the elbow (figure 16-20C). The main pressure point for the leg is the femoral artery. The pulsation can be felt at the groin (the front middle point of the upper leg, in the crease where the thigh joins the body) (figure 16-20D). When bleeding stops, slowly release pressure on the pressure point. Continue using direct pressure and elevation. If bleeding starts again, be ready to reapply pressure to the correct pressure point.

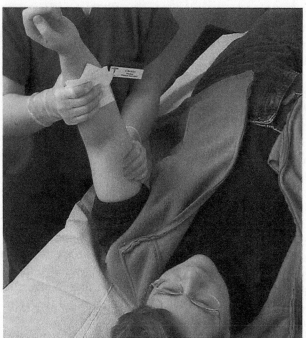

FIGURE 16-20C The main pressure point for the arm is the brachial artery. Pressure is applied to the artery only until the bleeding stops.

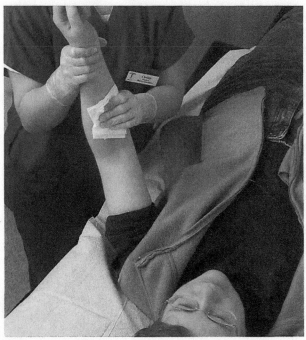

FIGURE 16-20B Continue to apply direct pressure while elevating the injured part above the level of the heart.

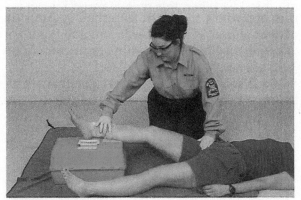

FIGURE 16-20D The main pressure point in the leg is the femoral artery. Pressure is applied while maintaining direct pressure to and elevation of the injured part.

After severe bleeding has been controlled, obtain medical help for the victim. Do not disturb any blood clots or remove the dressings that were used to control the bleeding, because this may result in additional bleeding. Make no attempt to clean the wound, because this too is likely to result in additional bleeding.

MINOR WOUNDS

In treating minor wounds that do not involve severe bleeding, prevention of infection is the first priority. Wash your hands thoroughly before treating the wound. Put on gloves to avoid contamination from blood or fluid draining from the wound. Use soap and water and sterile gauze, if possible, to wash the wound. Wipe in an outward direction, away from the wound. Discard the wipe after each use. Rinse the wound thoroughly with cool water. Use sterile gauze to gently blot the wound dry. Apply a sterile dressing or bandage. Watch for any signs of infection. Be sure to tell the victim to obtain medical help if any signs of infection appear.

Infection can develop in any wound. It is important to recognize the signs of infection and to seek medical help if they appear. Some signs and symptoms are swelling, heat, redness, pain, fever, pus, and red streaks leading from the wound. Prompt medical care is needed if any of these symptoms occur.

Tetanus bacteria can enter an open wound and lead to serious illness and death. Tetanus infection is most common in puncture wounds and wounds that involve damage to tissue underneath the skin. When this type of wound occurs, it is important to obtain information from the patient regarding his or her last tetanus shot and to get medical advice regarding protection in the form of a tetanus shot or booster.

With some wounds, objects can remain in the tissues or become embedded in the wound.

Examples of such objects include splinters, small pieces of glass, small stones, and other similar objects. If the object is at the surface of the skin, remove it gently with sterile tweezers or tweezers wiped clean with alcohol or a disinfectant. Any objects embedded in the tissues should be left in the skin and removed by a physician.

CLOSED WOUNDS

Closed wounds (those not involving breaks in the skin) can occur anywhere in the body as a result of injury. If the wound is a bruise, cold applications can be applied to reduce swelling. Other closed wounds can be extremely serious and cause internal bleeding that may lead to death. Signs and symptoms may include pain, tenderness, swelling, deformity, cold and clammy skin, rapid and weak pulse, a drop in blood pressure, uncontrolled restlessness, excessive thirst, vomited blood, or blood in the urine or feces. Get medical help for the victim as soon as possible. Check breathing, treat for shock, avoid unnecessary movement, and avoid giving any fluids or food to the victim.

SUMMARY

While caring for any victim with severe bleeding or wounds, always be alert for the signs of shock. Be prepared to treat shock while providing care to control bleeding and prevent infection in the wound.

At all times, remain calm while providing first aid. Reassure the victim. Obtain appropriate assistance or medical care as soon as possible in every case requiring additional care.

STUDENT: *Go to the workbook and complete the assignment sheet for 16:3, Providing First Aid for Bleeding and Wounds. Then return and continue with the procedure.*

PROCEDURE 16:3

Providing First Aid for Bleeding and Wounds

Equipment and Supplies

Sterile dressings and bandages, disposable gloves

Procedure

Severe Wounds

1. Follow the steps of priority care, if indicated.

   a. Check the scene. Move the victim only if absolutely necessary.

   b. Check the victim for consciousness and breathing.

   c. Call emergency medical services (EMS).

   d. Provide care to the victim.

2. To control severe bleeding, proceed as follows:

   a. If possible, put on gloves or wrap your hands in plastic wrap to provide a protective barrier while controlling bleeding. If this is not possible in an emergency, use thick layers of dressings and try to avoid contact of blood with your skin.

   b. Using your hand over a thick dressing or sterile gauze, apply pressure directly to the wound.

   c. Continue to apply pressure to the wound for approximately 5–10 minutes. Do *not* release the pressure to check whether the bleeding has stopped.

   d. If blood soaks through the first dressing, apply a second dressing on top of the first dressing, and continue to apply direct pressure.

   NOTE: If sterile gauze is *not* available, use clean material or a bare hand.

CAUTION: Do *not* disturb blood clots once they have formed. This will cause the bleeding to start again.

3. Elevate the injured part above the level of the victim's heart unless a fracture or broken bone is suspected.

   NOTE: This allows gravity to help stop the blood flow to the area.

   NOTE: Direct pressure and elevation are used together. Do *not* stop direct pressure while elevating the part.

4. To hold the dressings in place, apply a pressure bandage. Maintain direct pressure and elevation while applying the pressure bandage. To apply a pressure bandage, proceed as follows:

   a. Apply additional dressings over the dressings already on the wound.

   b. Use a roller bandage to hold the dressings in place by wrapping the roller bandage around the dressings. Use overlapping turns to cover the dressings and to hold them securely in place.

   c. Tie off the ends of the bandage by placing the tie directly over the dressings (figure 16-21).

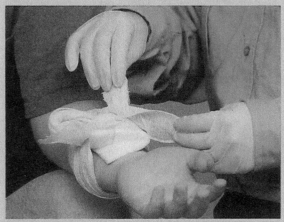

FIGURE 16-21 Tie the ends of the bandage directly over the dressings to secure a pressure bandage.

PROCEDURE 16:3

d. Make sure the pressure bandage is secure. Check a pulse site below the pressure bandage to make sure the bandage is not too tight. A pulse should be present and there should be no discoloration of the skin to indicate impaired circulation. If any signs of impaired circulation are present, loosen and replace the pressure bandage.

5. If the bleeding continues, it may be necessary to apply pressure to the appropriate pressure point. Continue using direct pressure and elevation, and apply pressure to the pressure point as follows:

a. If the wound is on the arm or hand, apply pressure to the brachial artery. Place the flat surface of your fingers (not your fingertips) against the inside of the victim's upper arm, approximately halfway between the elbow and axilla area. Position your thumb on the outside of the arm. Press your fingers toward your thumb to compress the brachial artery and decrease the supply of blood to the arm (refer to figure 16-20C).

b. If the wound is on the leg, place the flat surfaces of your fingers or the heel of one hand directly over the femoral artery where it passes over the pelvic bone. The position is on the front, middle part of the upper thigh (groin) where the leg joins the body. Straighten your arm and apply pressure to compress the femoral artery and to decrease the blood supply to the leg (refer to figure 16-20D).

6. When the bleeding stops, slowly release the pressure on the pressure point while continuing to use direct pressure and elevation. If the bleeding starts again, be ready to reapply pressure to the pressure point.

7. Obtain medical help for the victim as soon as possible. Severe bleeding is a life-threatening emergency.

8. While caring for any victim experiencing severe bleeding, be alert for the signs and symptoms of shock. Treat the victim for shock if any signs or symptoms are noted.

9. During treatment, constantly reassure the victim. Encourage the victim to remain calm by remaining calm yourself.

10. After controlling the bleeding, wash your hands as thoroughly and quickly as possible to avoid possible contamination from the blood. Wear gloves and use a disinfectant solution to wipe up any blood spills. Always wash your hands thoroughly after removing gloves.

Procedure
Minor Wounds

1. Wash hands thoroughly with soap and water. Put on gloves.

2. Use sterile gauze, soap, and water to wash the wound. Start at the center and wash in an outward direction. Discard the gauze after each pass.

3. Rinse the wound thoroughly with cool water to remove all of the soap.

4. Use sterile gauze to dry the wound. Blot it gently.

5. Apply a sterile dressing to the wound.

6. Caution the victim to look for signs of infection. Tell the victim to obtain medical care if any signs of infection appear.

7. If tetanus infection is possible (for example, in cases involving puncture wounds), tell the victim to contact a doctor regarding a tetanus shot.

CAUTION: Do *not* use any antiseptic solutions to clean the wound and do *not*

PROCEDURE 16:3

apply any substances to the wound unless specifically instructed to do so by a physician or your immediate supervisor.

8. Obtain medical help as soon as possible for any victim requiring additional care. Any victim who has particles embedded in a wound, risk for tetanus, severe bleeding, or other complications must be referred for medical care.

9. When care is complete, remove gloves and wash hands thoroughly.

Practice

Go to the workbook and use the evaluation sheet for 16:3, Providing First Aid for Bleeding and Wounds, to practice these procedures. When you believe you have mastered these skills, sign the sheet and give it to your instructor for further action.

✔ **Final Checkpoint** Using the criteria listed on the evaluation sheet, your instructor will grade your performance.

16:4 INFORMATION

Providing First Aid for Shock

INTRODUCTION

Shock is a state that can exist with any injury or illness requiring first aid. It is important that you are able to recognize it and provide treatment.

Shock, also called *hypoperfusion*, can be defined as "a clinical set of signs and symptoms associated with an inadequate supply of blood to body organs, especially the brain and heart." If it is not treated, shock can lead to death, even when a victim's injuries or illness might not themselves be fatal. After just 4–6 minutes of hypoperfusion, brains cells are damaged irreversibly.

CAUSES OF SHOCK

Many different things can cause the victim to experience shock: **hemorrhage** (excessive loss of blood); excessive pain; infection; heart attack; stroke; poisoning by chemicals, drugs, or gases; lack of oxygen; psychological trauma; and dehydration (loss of body fluids) from burns, vomiting, or diarrhea. The eight main types of shock are shown in Table 16-1. All types of shock impair

circulation and decrease the supply of oxygen to body cells, tissues, and organs.

SIGNS AND SYMPTOMS

When shock occurs, the body attempts to increase blood flow to the brain, heart, and vital organs by reducing blood flow to other body parts. This can lead to the following signs and symptoms that indicate shock:

◆ Skin is pale or cyanotic (bluish gray) in color. Check the nail beds and the mucous membrane around the mouth.

◆ Skin is cool to the touch.

◆ **Diaphoresis**, or excessive perspiration, may result in a wet, clammy feeling when the skin is touched.

◆ Pulse is rapid, weak, and difficult to feel. Check the pulse at one of the carotid arteries in the neck.

◆ Respirations are rapid, shallow, and may be irregular.

◆ Blood pressure is very low or below normal, and may not be obtainable.

◆ Victim experiences general weakness. As shock progresses, the victim becomes listless

TABLE 16-1 Types of Shock

TYPE OF SHOCK	CAUSE	DESCRIPTION
Anaphylactic	Hypersensitive or allergic reaction to a substance such as food, medications, insect stings or bites, or snake bites	Body releases histamine causing vasodilation (blood vessels get larger) Blood pressure drops and less blood goes to body cells Urticaria (hives) and respiratory distress may occur
Cardiogenic	Damage to heart muscle from heart attack or cardiac arrest	Heart cannot effectively pump blood to body cells
Hemorrhagic	Severe bleeding or loss of blood plasma	Decrease in blood volume causes blood pressure to drop Decreased blood flow to body cells
Metabolic	Loss of body fluid from severe vomiting, diarrhea, or a heat illness Disruption in acid–base balance as occurs in diabetes	Decreased amount of fluid causes dehydration and disruption in normal acid–base balance of body Blood pressure drops and less blood circulates to body cells
Neurogenic	Injury and trauma to brain and/or spinal cord	Nervous system loses ability to control the size of blood vessels Blood vessels dilate and blood pressure drops Decreased blood flow to body cells
Psychogenic	Emotional distress such as anger, fear, or grief	Emotional response causes sudden dilation of blood vessels Blood pools in areas away from the brain Some individuals faint
Respiratory	Trauma to respiratory tract Respiratory distress or arrest (chronic disease, choking)	Interferes with exchange of oxygen and carbon dioxide between lungs and bloodstream Insufficient oxygen supply for body cells
Septic	Acute infection (toxic shock syndrome)	Poisons or toxins in blood cause vasodilation Blood pressure drops Less oxygen to body cells

and confused. Eventually, the victim loses consciousness.

◆ Victim experiences anxiety and extreme restlessness.

◆ Victim may experience excessive thirst, nausea, and/or vomiting.

◆ Victim may complain of blurred vision. As shock progresses, the victim's eyes may appear sunken and have a vacant or confused expression. The pupils may dilate or become large.

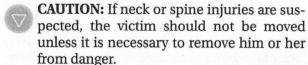

TREATMENT FOR SHOCK

It is essential to get medical help for the victim as soon as possible because shock is a life-threatening condition. Treatment for shock is directed toward (1) eliminating the cause of shock; (2) improving circulation, especially to the brain and heart; (3) providing an adequate oxygen supply; and (4) maintaining body temperature. Some of the basic principles for treatment are as follows:

◆ Reduce the effects of or eliminate the cause of shock: control bleeding, provide oxygen if available, ease pain through position change, and/or provide emotional support.

◆ The position for treating shock must be based on the victim's injuries.

▽ **CAUTION:** If neck or spine injuries are suspected, the victim should not be moved unless it is necessary to remove him or her from danger.

The best position for treating shock is usually to keep the victim lying flat on the back, because this improves circulation. Raising the feet and legs approximately 12 inches can also provide additional blood for the heart and brain. However, if the victim is vomiting or has bleeding and injuries of the jaw or mouth, the victim should be positioned on the side to prevent him or her from choking on blood and/or vomitus. If a victim is experiencing breathing problems, it may be necessary to raise the victim's head and shoulders to make breathing easier. If the victim has a *head* (not neck) injury and has difficulty breathing, the victim should be positioned lying flat or with the head raised slightly. It is important to position the victim based on the injury or illness involved.

♦ Cover the patient with blankets or additional clothing to prevent chilling or exposure to the cold. Blankets may also be placed between the ground and the victim. However, it is important to avoid overheating the victim. If the skin is very warm to the touch and perspiration is noted, remove some of the blankets or coverings.

♦ Avoid giving the victim anything to eat or drink. If the victim complains of excessive thirst, a wet cloth can be used to provide some comfort by moistening the lips and mouth.

Remember that it is important to look for signs of shock while providing first aid for any injury or illness. Provide care that will reduce the effect of shock. Obtain medical help for the victim as soon as possible.

STUDENT: *Go to the workbook and complete the assignment sheet for 16:4, Providing First Aid for Shock. Then return and continue with the procedure.*

PROCEDURE 16:4

Providing First Aid for Shock

Equipment and Supplies

Blankets, watch with second hand (optional), disposable gloves

Procedure

1. Follow the steps of priority care, if indicated.

   a. Check the scene. Move the victim only if absolutely necessary.

   b. Check the victim for consciousness and breathing.

   c. Call emergency medical services (EMS).

   d. Provide care to the victim.

   e. Control severe bleeding.

   CAUTION: If possible, wear gloves or use a protective barrier while controlling bleeding.

2. Obtain medical help for the victim as soon as possible. Call or send someone to obtain help.

3. Observe the victim for any signs of shock. Look for a pale or cyanotic (bluish) color to the skin. Touch the skin and note if it is cool, moist, or clammy to the touch. Note diaphoresis, or excessive perspiration. Check the pulse to see if it is rapid, weak, or irregular. If you are unable to feel a radial pulse, check the carotid pulse. Check the respirations to see if they are rapid, weak, irregular, shallow, or labored. If equipment is available, check blood pressure to see if it is low. Observe the victim for signs of weakness, apathy, confusion, or consciousness. Note if the victim is nauseated or vomiting, complaining of excessive thirst, restless or anxious, or complaining of blurred vision. Examine the eyes for a sunken, vacant, or confused appearance, and dilated pupils.

4. Try to reduce the effects or eliminate the cause of shock:

   a. Control bleeding by applying pressure at the site.

   b. Provide oxygen, if possible.

   c. Attempt to ease pain through position changes and comfort measures.

   d. Give emotional support.

PROCEDURE 16:4

5. Position the victim based on the injuries or illness present.

   a. If an injury of the neck or spine is present or suspected, do not move the victim.

   b. If the victim has bleeding and injuries to the jaw or mouth, or is vomiting, position the victim's body on either side. This allows fluids, vomitus, and/or blood to drain and prevents the airway from becoming blocked by these fluids.

   c. If the victim is having difficulty breathing, position the victim on the back, but raise the head and shoulders slightly to aid breathing.

   d. If the victim has a head injury, position the victim lying flat or with the head raised slightly.

   NOTE: Never allow the head to be positioned lower than the rest of the body.

   e. If none of these conditions exist, position the victim lying flat on the back. To improve circulation, raise the feet and legs approximately 12 inches (figure 16-22). If raising the legs causes pain or leads to difficult breathing, however, lower the legs to the flat position.

   CAUTION: Do not raise the legs if the victim has head, neck, or back injuries, or if there are possible fractures of the hips or legs.

   f. If in doubt on how to position a victim according to the injuries involved, keep the victim lying down flat or in the position in which you found him or her. Avoid any unnecessary movement.

6. Place enough blankets or coverings on the victim to prevent chilling. Sometimes, a blanket can be placed between the victim and the ground. Avoid overheating the victim.

7. Do not give the victim anything to eat or drink. If the victim complains of excessive thirst, use a moist cloth to wet the lips, tongue, and inside of the mouth.

8. Constantly reassure the victim. Encourage the victim to remain calm by remaining calm yourself.

9. Observe and provide care to the victim until medical help is obtained.

10. Replace all equipment used. Wash hands.

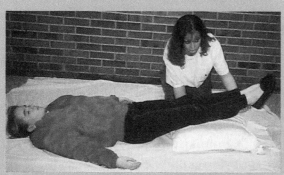

FIGURE 16-22 Position a shock victim flat on the back and elevate the feet and legs approximately 12 inches. Do *not* use this position if the victim has a neck, spinal, head, or jaw injury, or if the victim is having difficulty breathing.

Practice

Go to the workbook and use the evaluation sheet for 16:4, Providing First Aid for Shock, to practice this procedure. When you believe you have mastered this skill, sign the sheet and give it to your instructor for further action.

✔ **Final Checkpoint** Using the criteria listed on the evaluation sheet, your instructor will grade your performance.

16:5 INFORMATION

Providing First Aid for Poisoning

INTRODUCTION

Poisoning can occur anywhere, anytime—not only in health care settings, but also in your personal life. **Poisoning** can happen to any individual, regardless of age. It can be caused by ingesting (swallowing) various substances, inhaling poisonous gases, injecting substances, or contacting the skin with poison. Any substance that causes a harmful reaction when applied or ingested can be called a poison. Immediate action is necessary for any poisoning victim. Treatment varies depending on the type of poison, the injury involved, and the method of contact.

If the poisoning victim is unconscious, check for breathing. Provide artificial respiration if the victim is not breathing. Obtain medical help as soon as possible. If the unconscious victim is breathing, position the victim on his or her side so fluids can drain from the mouth. Obtain medical help quickly.

INGESTION POISONING

If a poison has been swallowed, immediate care must be provided before the poison can be absorbed into the body. Basic steps of first aid include:

- Call a poison control center (PCC) or a physician immediately. If you cannot contact a PCC, call emergency medical services (EMS). Most areas have poison control centers that provide information on specific antidotes and treatment.

- Save the label or container of the substance taken so this information can be given to the PCC or physician.

- Calculate or estimate how much was taken and the time at which the poisoning occurred.

- If the victim vomits, save a sample of the vomited material.

- If the PCC tells you to induce vomiting, get the victim to vomit. To induce vomiting, tickle the back of the victim's throat or give the victim warm saltwater to drink. In some cases, the PCC

may recommend giving syrup of ipecac followed by a glass of water. Recent studies have shown that syrup of ipecac can cause dehydration and confusion, so it should only be given if recommended by the PCC or a physician. Follow dosage recommended on bottle. Syrup of ipecac is available in most drug stores and can be kept in a first aid kit for poisoning victims.

- **CAUTION:** Vomiting must *not* be induced in unconscious victims, victims who swallowed an acid or alkali, victims who swallowed petroleum products, victims who are convulsing, or victims who have burns on the lips and mouth.

- Activated charcoal may be recommended by the PCC to bind to the poison so it is not absorbed into the body. Activated charcoal should only be given to victims who are conscious and able to swallow. It is available in most drug stores. The directions on the bottle should be followed to determine the correct dosage.

INHALATION POISONING

If poisoning is caused by inhalation of dangerous gases, the victim must be removed immediately from the area before being treated. A commonly inhaled poison is carbon monoxide. It is odorless, colorless, and very difficult to detect. Basic steps of first aid include:

- Before entering the danger area, take a deep breath of fresh air and do *not* breathe the gas while you are removing the victim from the area.

- After rescuing the victim, immediately check for breathing.

- Provide artificial respiration if needed.

- Obtain medical help immediately; death may occur very quickly with this type of poisoning.

CONTACT POISONING

If poisoning is caused by chemicals or poisons coming in contact with the victim's skin, care for the victim includes:

- Use large amounts of water to wash the skin for at least 15–20 minutes to dilute the substance and remove it from the skin.

♦ Remove any clothing and jewelry that contain the substance.

♦ Call a PCC or physician for additional information.

♦ Obtain medical help as soon as possible for burns or injuries that may result from contact with the poison.

Contact with a poisonous plant such as poison ivy, oak, or sumac can cause a serious skin reaction if not treated immediately. Basic steps of first aid include:

♦ Wash the area thoroughly with soap and water

♦ If a rash or weeping sores develop after 2–3 days, lotions such as Calamine or Caladryl, or a paste made from baking soda and water may help relieve the discomfort.

♦ If the condition is severe and affects large areas of the body or face, obtain medical help.

INJECTION POISONING

Injection poisoning occurs when an insect, spider, or snake bites or stings an individual. If an arm or leg is affected, position the affected area below the level of the heart. For an insect sting, first aid treatment includes:

♦ Remove any embedded stinger by scraping the stinger away from the skin with the edge of a rigid card, such as a credit card, or a tongue depressor. Do not use tweezers because tweezers can puncture the venom sac attached to the stinger, injecting more poison into body tissues.

♦ Wash the area well with soap and water.

♦ Apply a sterile dressing and a cold pack to reduce swelling.

If a tick is embedded in the skin, first aid treatment includes:

♦ Use tweezers to slowly pull the tick out of the skin.

♦ Wash the area thoroughly with soap and water.

♦ Apply an antiseptic.

♦ Watch for signs of infection.

♦ Obtain medical help if needed.

Ticks can cause Rocky Mountain spotted fever or Lyme disease, dangerous diseases if untreated.

For a snakebite or spider bite, first aid treatment includes:

♦ Wash the wound.

♦ Immobilize the injured area, positioning it lower than the heart, if possible.

♦ Do *not* cut the wound or apply a tourniquet.

♦ Monitor the breathing of the victim and give artificial respiration if necessary.

♦ Obtain medical help for the victim as soon as possible.

For any type of injection poisoning, watch for allergic reaction in all victims (figure 16-23). Signs and symptoms of allergic reaction include redness and swelling at the site, itching, hives, pain, swelling of the throat, difficult or labored breathing, dizziness, and a change in the level of consciousness. Maintain respirations and obtain medical help as quickly as possible for the victim who experiences an allergic reaction.

SUMMARY

In all poisoning victims, observe for signs of anaphylactic shock. Treat the victim for shock, if necessary. Try to remain calm and confident while providing first aid for poisoning victims. Reassure the victim as needed. Act quickly and in an organized, efficient manner.

STUDENT: *Go to the workbook and complete the assignment sheet for 16:5, Providing First Aid for Poisoning. Then return and continue with the procedure.*

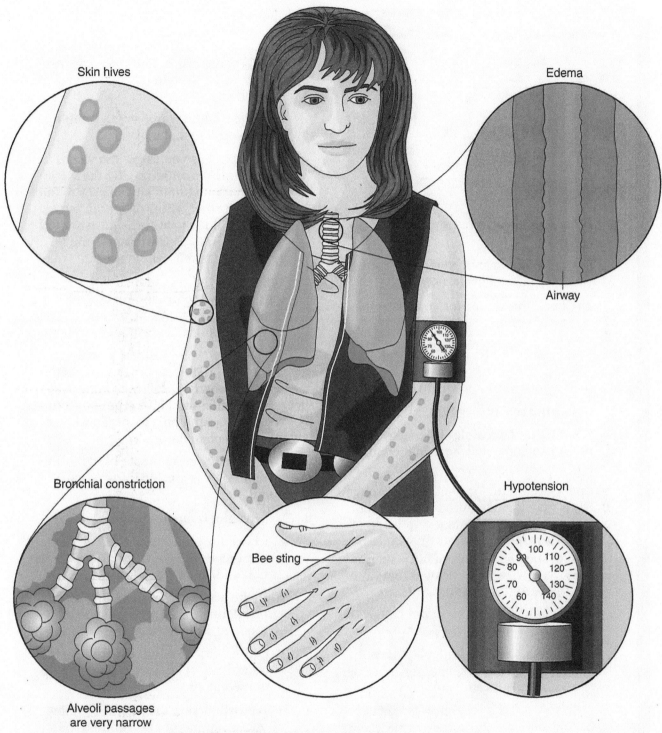

Skin hives

Edema

Airway

Bronchial constriction

Hypotension

Bee sting

Alveoli passages
are very narrow

FIGURE 16-23 Watch for allergic reactions in all poisoning victims.

PROCEDURE 16:5

Providing First Aid for Poisoning

Equipment and Supplies

Telephone, disposable gloves

Procedure

1. Follow the steps of priority care, if indicated:

   a. Check the scene. Move the victim only if absolutely necessary.

   b. Check the victim for consciousness and breathing.

   c. Call emergency medical services (EMS).

   d. Provide care to the victim.

   e. Control severe bleeding.

   CAUTION: If possible, wear gloves or use a protective barrier while controlling bleeding.

2. Check the victim for signs of poisoning. Signs may include burns on the lips or mouth, odor, a container of poison, or presence of the poisonous substance on the victim or in the victim's mouth. Information may also be obtained from the victim or from an observer.

3. If the victim is conscious, not convulsing, and has swallowed a poison:

   a. Try to determine the type of poison, how much was taken, and when the poison was taken. Look for the container near the victim.

   b. Call a poison control center (PCC) or physician immediately for specific information on how to treat the poisoning victim. Provide as much information as possible.

   c. Follow the instructions received from the PCC. Obtain medical help if needed.

   d. If the victim vomits, save a sample of the vomited material.

4. If the PCC tells you to get the victim to vomit, induce vomiting. Give the victim warm salt water or tickle the back of the victim's throat. Syrup of ipecac is also used to induce vomiting, but it should not be given to a victim unless the PCC or a physician tells you to use it.

   CAUTION: Do *not* induce vomiting if the victim is unconscious or convulsing, has burns on the lips or mouth, or has swallowed an acid, alkali, or petroleum product.

5. If the PCC tells you to give the victim activated charcoal, follow the directions on the container. Make sure the victim is conscious and able to swallow before giving the charcoal.

   NOTE: Activated charcoal binds to the poison so it is not absorbed into the body.

6. If the victim is unconscious:

   a. Check for breathing. If the victim is not breathing, give artificial respiration and/or CPR as needed.

   b. If the victim is breathing, position the victim on his or her side to allow fluids to drain from the mouth.

   c. Call a PCC or physician for specific treatment. Obtain medical help immediately.

   d. If possible, save the poison container and a sample of any vomited material. Check with any observers to find out what was taken, how much was taken, and when the poison was taken.

7. If chemicals or poisons have splashed on the victim's skin, wash the area thoroughly with large amounts of water.

PROCEDURE 16:5

Remove any clothing and jewelry containing the substance. If a large area of the body is affected, a shower, tub, or garden hose may be used to rinse the skin. Obtain medical help immediately for burns or injuries caused by the poison.

8. If the victim has come in contact with a poisonous plant such as poison ivy, oak, or sumac, wash the area of contact thoroughly with soap and water. Remove any contaminated clothing. If a rash or weeping sores develop in the next few days after exposure, lotions such as Calamine or Caladryl, or a paste made from baking soda and water, may help relieve the discomfort. If the condition is severe and affects large areas of the body or face, obtain medical help.

9. If the victim has inhaled poisonous gas, do not endanger your life by trying to treat the victim in the area of the gas. Take a deep breath of fresh air before entering the area and hold your breath while you remove the victim from the area. When the victim is in a safe area, check for breathing. Provide artificial respiration and/or CPR as needed. Obtain medical help immediately.

10. If poisoning is caused by injection from an insect bite or sting or a snakebite, proceed as follows:

    a. If an arm or leg is affected, position the affected area below the level of the heart.

    b. For an insect bite, remove any embedded stinger by scraping it off with an object like a credit card. Wash the area well with soap and water. Apply a sterile dressing and a cold pack to reduce swelling.

    c. If a tick is embedded in the skin, use tweezers to gently pull the tick out of the skin. Wash the area thoroughly with soap and water, and apply an antiseptic. Obtain medical help if needed.

    d. For a snakebite, wash the wound. Immobilize the injured area, positioning it lower than the heart if possible. Monitor the breathing of the victim and give artificial respiration if necessary. Obtain medical help for the victim as soon as possible.

    e. Watch for the signs and symptoms of allergic reaction in all victims. Signs and symptoms of allergic reaction include redness and swelling at the site, itching, hives (figure 16-24), pain, swelling of the throat, difficult or labored breathing, dizziness, and a change in the level of consciousness. Maintain respirations and obtain medical help as quickly as possible for the victim experiencing an allergic reaction.

11. Observe for signs of anaphylactic shock while treating any poisoning victim. Treat for shock as necessary.

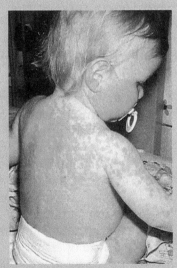

FIGURE 16-24 Hives are a common sign of an allergic reaction. *(Courtesy of Robert A. Silverman, MD, Clinical Associate Professor, Department of Pediatrics, Georgetown University, Georgetown, MD)*

PROCEDURE 16:5

12. Remain calm while treating the victim. Reassure the victim.

13. Always obtain medical help for any poisoning victim. Some poisons may have delayed reactions. Always keep the telephone numbers of a PCC and other sources of medical assistance in a convenient location so you will be prepared to provide first aid for poisoning.

14. Wash hands thoroughly after providing care.

Practice

Go to the workbook and use the evaluation sheet for 16:5, Providing First Aid for Poisoning, to practice this procedure. When you believe you have mastered this skill, sign the sheet and give it to your instructor for further action.

✓ **Final Checkpoint** Using the criteria listed on the evaluation sheet, your instructor will grade your performance.

16:6 INFORMATION

Providing First Aid for Burns

TYPES OF BURNS

A **burn** is an injury that can be caused by fire, heat, chemical agents, radiation, and/or electricity. Burns are classified as either superficial, partial thickness, or full thickness (figure 16-25). Characteristics of each type of burn are as follows:

◆ *Superficial, or first-degree, burn*: This is the least severe type of burn. It involves only the top layer of skin, the epidermis, and usually heals in 5–6 days without permanent scarring. The skin is usually reddened or discolored. There may be some mild swelling, and the victim feels pain. Three common causes are overexposure to the sun (sunburn), brief contact with hot objects or steam, and exposure of the skin to a weak acid or alkali.

◆ *Partial-thickness, or second-degree, burn*: This type of burn involves injury to the top layers of skin, including both the epidermis and dermis. A blister or vesicle forms. The skin is red or has a mottled appearance. Swelling usually occurs, and the surface of the skin frequently appears to be wet. This is a painful burn and

may take 3–4 weeks to heal. Frequent causes include excessive exposure to the sun, a sunlamp, or artificial radiation; contact with hot or boiling liquids; and contact with fire.

◆ *Full-thickness, or third-degree, burn*: This is the most severe type of burn and involves injury to all layers of the skin plus the underlying tissue. The area involved has a white or charred appearance. This type of burn can be either extremely painful or, if nerve endings are destroyed, relatively painless. Third-degree burns can be life-threatening because of fluid loss, infection, and shock. Frequent causes include exposure to fire or flames, prolonged contact with hot objects, contact with electricity, and immersion in hot or boiling liquids.

TREATMENT

First aid treatment for burns is directed toward removing the source of heat, cooling the affected skin area, covering the burn, relieving pain, observing and treating for shock, and preventing infection. Medical treatment is not usually required for superficial and mild partial-thickness burns. However, medical care should be obtained if more than 15 percent of the surface of an adult's body is burned (10 percent in a child).

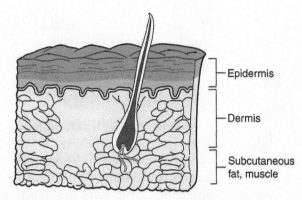

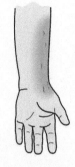

Epidermis

Dermis

Subcutaneous fat, muscle

Skin red, dry

Superficial, first degree

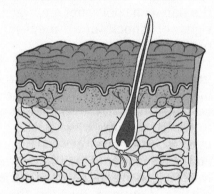

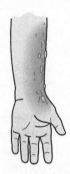

Blistered, skin moist, pink or red

Partial thickness, second degree

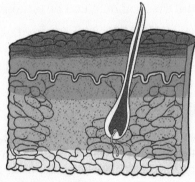

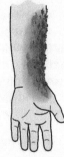

Charring, skin black, brown, red

Full thickness, third degree

FIGURE 16-25 Types of burns

The rule of nines is used to calculate the percentage of body surface burned (figure 16-26). Medical care should also be obtained if the burns affect the face or respiratory tract; if the victim has difficulty breathing; if burns cover more than one body part; if the victim has a partial-thickness burn and is under 5 or over 60 years of age; or if the burns resulted from chemicals, explosions, or electricity. All victims with full-thickness burns should receive medical care.

Superficial and Mild Partial-Thickness Burns

The main treatment for superficial and mild partial-thickness burns is to cool the area by flushing it with large amounts of cool water. Do *not* use ice or ice water on burns because doing so causes the body to lose heat. After the pain subsides, use dry, sterile gauze to blot the area dry. Apply a dry, sterile dressing to prevent infec-

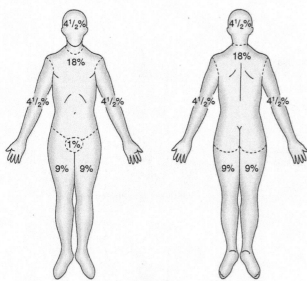

FIGURE 16-26 The *rule of nines* is used to calculate the percentage of body surface burned.

tion. If nonadhesive dressings are available, it is best to use them because they will not stick to the injured area. If possible, elevate the affected part to reduce swelling caused by inflammation. If necessary, obtain medical help.

 CAUTION: Do *not* apply cotton, tissues, ointment, powders, oils, grease, butter, or any other substances to the burned area unless you are instructed to do so by a physician or your immediate supervisor. Do *not* break or open any blisters that form on burns because doing so will just cause an open wound that is prone to infection.

Severe Partial-Thickness and Full-Thickness Burns

Call for medical help immediately if the victim has severe partial-thickness or full-thickness burns. Cover the burned areas with thick, sterile dressings. Elevate the hands or feet if they are burned. If the feet or legs are burned, do *not* allow the victim to walk. If particles of clothing are attached to the burned areas, do *not* attempt to remove these particles. Watch the victim closely for signs of respiratory distress and/or shock.

Provide artificial respiration and treatment for shock, as necessary. Watch the victim closely until medical help arrives.

Chemical Burns

For burns caused by chemicals splashing on the skin, use large amounts of water to flush the affected areas for 15–30 minutes or until medical help arrives. Gently remove any clothing, socks and shoes, or jewelry that contains the chemical to minimize the area injured. Continue flushing the skin with cool water and watch the victim for signs of shock until medical help can be obtained.

If the *eyes* have been burned by chemicals or irritating gases, flush the eyes with large amounts of water for at least 15–30 minutes or until medical help arrives. If only one eye is injured, be sure to tilt the victim's head in the direction of the injury so the injured eye can be properly flushed. Start at the inner corner of the eye and allow the water to run over the surface of the eye and to the outside. Continue flushing the eye with cool water and watch the victim for signs of shock until medical help can be obtained.

 CAUTION: Make sure that the water (or remaining chemical) does not enter the *uninjured* eye.

SUMMARY

Loss of body fluids (dehydration) can occur very quickly with severe burns, so shock is frequently noted in burn victims. Be alert for any signs of shock and treat the burn victim for shock immediately.

Remain calm while treating the burn victim. Reassure the victim. Obtain medical help as quickly as possible for any burn victim requiring medical assistance.

STUDENT: *Go to the workbook and complete the assignment sheet for 16:6, Providing First Aid for Burns. Then return and continue with the procedure.*

PROCEDURE 16:6

Providing First Aid for Burns

Equipment and Supplies

Water, sterile dressings, disposable gloves

Procedure

1. Follow the priorities of care, if indicated:

   a. Check the scene. Move the victim only if absolutely necessary.

   b. Check the victim for consciousness and breathing.

   c. Call emergency medical services (EMS) if necessary.

   d. Provide care to the victim.

   e. Check for bleeding. Control severe bleeding.

   CAUTION: If possible, wear gloves or use a protective barrier while controlling bleeding.

2. Check the burned area carefully to determine the type of burn. A reddened or discolored area is usually a superficial, or first-degree, burn. If the skin is wet, red, swollen, painful, and blistered, the burn is usually a partial-thickness, or second-degree, burn (figure 16-27A). If the skin is white or charred and there is destruction of tissue, the burn is a full-thickness, or third-degree, burn (figure 16-27B).

   NOTE: Victims can have more than one type of burn at one time. Treat for the most severe type of burn present.

3. For a superficial or mild partial-thickness burn:

   a. Cool the burn by flushing it with large amounts of cool water. If this is not possible, apply clean or sterile cloths that are cold and wet. Continue

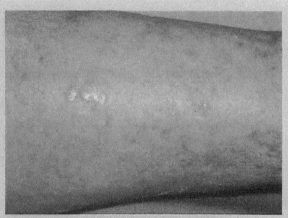

FIGURE 16-27A The skin is wet, red, swollen, painful, and blistered when a partial-thickness burn is present. *(Courtesy of the Phoenix Society of Burn Survivors, Inc.)*

applying cold water until the pain subsides.

   b. Use sterile gauze to gently blot the injured area dry.

   c. Apply dry, sterile dressings to the burned area. If possible, use nonadhesive (nonstick) dressings, because they will not stick to the burn.

   d. If blisters are present, do *not* break or open them.

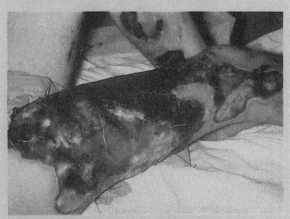

FIGURE 16-27B A full-thickness burn destroys or affects all layers of the skin plus fat, muscle, bone, and nerve tissue. The skin is white or charred in appearance. *(Courtesy of the Phoenix Society of Burn Survivors, Inc.)*

PROCEDURE 16:6

e. If possible, elevate the burned area to reduce swelling caused by inflammation.

f. Obtain medical help for burns to the face, or if burns cover more than 15 percent of the surface of an adult's body or 10 percent of the surface of a child's body. If the victim is having difficulty breathing, or any other distress is noted, obtain medical help.

g. Do *not* apply any cotton, ointment, powders, grease, butter, or similar substances to the burned area.

NOTE: These substances may increase the possibility of infection.

4. For a severe partial-thickness or any full-thickness burn:

a. Call for medical help immediately.

b. Use thick, sterile dressings to cover the injured areas.

c. Do *not* attempt to remove any particles of clothing that have stuck to the burned areas.

d. If the hands and arms or legs and feet are affected, elevate these areas.

e. If the victim has burns on the face or is experiencing difficulty in breathing, elevate the head.

f. Watch the victim closely for signs of shock and provide care if necessary.

5. For a burn caused by a chemical splashing on the skin:

a. Using large amounts of water, immediately flush the area for 15–30 minutes or until medical help arrives.

b. Remove any articles of clothing, socks and shoes, or jewelry contaminated by the substance.

c. Continue flushing the area with large amounts of cool water.

d. Obtain medical help immediately.

6. If the eye has been burned by chemicals or irritating gases:

a. If the victim is wearing contact lenses or glasses, ask him or her to remove them quickly.

b. Tilt the victim's head toward the injured side.

c. Hold the eyelid of the injured eye open. Pour cool water from the inner part of the eye (the part closest to the nose) toward the outer part (figure 16-28).

d. Use cool water to irrigate the eye for 15–30 minutes or until medical help arrives.

CAUTION: Take care that the water or chemicals do not enter the uninjured eye. ·

e. Obtain medical help immediately.

7. Observe for the signs of shock in all burn victims. Treat for shock as necessary.

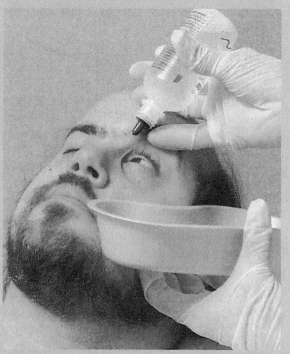

FIGURE 16-28 To irrigate an eye, hold the eyelid open and irrigate from the inner part of the eye toward the outer part.

PROCEDURE 16:6

8. Reassure the victim as you are providing treatment. Remain calm and encourage the victim to remain calm.

9. Obtain medical help immediately for any burn victim with extensive burns, full-thickness burns, burns to the face, signs of shock, respiratory distress, eye burns, and/or chemical burns to the skin.

10. Wash hands thoroughly after providing care.

Practice

Go to the workbook and use the evaluation sheet for 16:6, Providing First Aid for Burns, to practice this procedure. When you believe you have mastered this skill, sign the sheet and give it to your instructor for further action.

✔ **Final Checkpoint** Using the criteria listed on the evaluation sheet, your instructor will grade your performance.

16:7 INFORMATION

Providing First Aid for Heat Exposure

Excessive exposure to heat or high external temperatures can lead to a life-threatening emergency (figure 16-29). Overexposure to heat can cause a chemical imbalance in the body that can eventually lead to death. Harmful reactions can occur when water or salt are lost through perspiration or when the body cannot eliminate excess heat.

Heat cramps are caused by exposure to heat. They are muscle pains and spasms that result from the loss of water and salt through perspiration. Firm pressure applied to the cramped muscle will provide relief from the discomfort. The victim should rest and move to a cooler area. In addition, small sips of water or an electrolyte solution, such as sport drinks, can be given to the victim.

Heat exhaustion occurs when a victim is exposed to heat and experiences a loss of fluids through sweating. Signs and symptoms include pale and clammy skin, profuse perspiration (diaphoresis), fatigue or tiredness, weakness, headache, muscle cramps, nausea and/or vomiting, and dizziness and/or fainting. Body temperature is about normal or just slightly elevated. It is important to treat heat exhaustion as quickly as

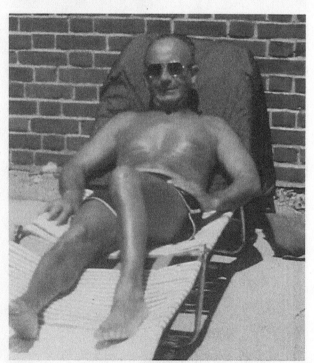

FIGURE 16-29 Excessive exposure to heat or high external temperatures can lead to a life-threatening emergency. *(Courtesy of the Phoenix Society of Burn Survivors, Inc.)*

possible. If it is not treated, it can develop into heat stroke. Treatment methods include moving the victim to a cooler area whenever possible; loosening or removing excessive clothing; applying cool, wet cloths; laying the victim down and elevating the victim's feet 12 inches; and giving the victim small sips of cool water, approximately 4 ounces every 15 minutes if the victim is alert and conscious. If the victim vomits, develops shock, or experiences respiratory distress, medical help should be obtained immediately.

Heat stroke is caused by prolonged exposure to high temperatures. It is a medical emergency. The body is unable to eliminate the excess heat, and internal body temperature rises to 105°F (40.6°C) or higher. Normal body defenses such as the sweating mechanism no longer function. Signs and symptoms in addition to the high body temperature include red, hot, and dry skin. The pulse is usually rapid, but may remain strong. The victim may lose consciousness. Treatment is geared primarily toward ways of cooling the body quickly, because a high body temperature can cause convulsions and/or death in a very short period of time. The victim can be placed in a tub of cool water, or the skin can be sponged with cool water. Ice or cold packs can be placed on the victim's wrists, ankles, in each axillary (armpit) area, and in the groin. Be alert for signs of shock at all times. Obtain medical help immediately.

After victims have recovered from any condition caused by heat exposure, they must be warned to avoid abnormally warm or hot temperatures for several days. They should also be encouraged to drink sufficient amounts of water and/or electrolyte solutions.

STUDENT: *Go to the workbook and complete the assignment sheet for 16:7, Providing First Aid for Heat Exposure. Then return and continue with the procedure.*

PROCEDURE 16:7

Providing First Aid for Heat Exposure

Equipment and Supplies

Water, wash cloths or small towels

Procedure

1. Follow the priorities of care, if indicated:

   a. Check the scene. Move the victim only if absolutely necessary.

   b. Check the victim for consciousness and breathing.

   c. Call emergency medical services (EMS) if necessary.

   d. Provide care to the victim.

   e. Check for bleeding. Control severe bleeding.

   CAUTION: If possible, wear gloves or use a protective barrier while controlling bleeding.

2. Observe the victim closely for signs and symptoms of heat exposure. Information may also be obtained directly from the victim or from observers. If the victim has been exposed to heat or has been exercising strenuously, and is complaining of muscular pain or spasm, he or she is probably experiencing heat cramps. If the victim has close-to-normal body temperature but has pale and clammy skin, is perspiring excessively, and complains of nausea, headache, weakness, dizziness, or fatigue, he or she is probably experiencing heat exhaustion. If body temperature is high (105°F, or 40.6°C, or higher); skin is red, dry, and hot; and the victim is weak or unconscious, he or she is experiencing heat stroke.

3. If the victim has heat cramps:

   a. Use your hand to apply firm pressure to the cramped muscle(s). This helps relieve the spasms.

   b. Encourage relaxation. Allow the victim to lie down in a cool area, if possible.

   c. If the victim is alert and conscious and is not nauseated or vomiting, give him or her small sips of cool

PROCEDURE 16:7

water or an electrolyte solution such as a sport drink. Encourage the victim to drink approximately 4 ounces every 15 minutes.

   d. If the heat cramps continue or get worse, obtain medical help.

4. If the victim has heat exhaustion:

   a. Move the victim to a cool area, if possible. An air-conditioned room is ideal, but a fan can also help circulate air and cool the victim.

   b. Help the victim lie down flat on the back. Elevate the victim's feet and legs 12 inches.

   c. Loosen any tight clothing. Remove excessive clothing such as jackets and sweaters.

   d. Apply cool, wet cloths to the victim's face.

   e. If the victim is conscious and is not nauseated or vomiting, give him or her small sips of cool water or an electrolyte solution such as a sport drink. Encourage the victim to drink approximately 4 ounces every 15 minutes.

   f. If the victim complains of nausea and/or vomits, discontinue the water. Obtain medical help.

5. If the victim has heat stroke:

   a. Immediately move the victim to a cool area, if at all possible.

   b. Remove excessive clothing.

   c. Sponge the bare skin with cool water, or place ice or cold packs on the victim's wrists, ankles, and in the axillary and groin areas. The victim can also be placed in a tub of cool water to lower body temperature.

 CAUTION: Watch that the victim's head is not submerged in water. If the victim is unconscious, you may need assistance to place him or her in the tub.

   d. If vomiting occurs, position the victim on his or her side. Watch for signs of difficulty in breathing and provide care as indicated.

   e. Obtain medical help immediately. This is a life-threatening emergency.

6. Shock can develop quickly in all victims of heat exposure. Be alert for the signs of shock and treat as necessary.

 CAUTION: Obtain medical help for heat cramps that do not subside, heat exhaustion with signs of shock or vomiting, and *all* heat stroke victims as soon as possible.

7. Reassure the victim as you are providing treatment. Remain calm.

8. Wash hands thoroughly after providing care.

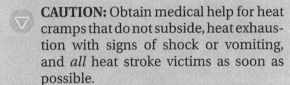

Practice

Go to the workbook and use the evaluation sheet for 16:7, Providing First Aid for Heat Exposure, to practice this procedure. When you believe you have mastered this skill, sign the sheet and give it to your instructor for further action.

✔ **Final Checkpoint** Using the criteria listed on the evaluation sheet, your instructor will grade your performance.

16:8 INFORMATION

Providing First Aid for Cold Exposure

Exposure to cold external temperatures can cause body tissues to freeze and body processes to slow. If treatment is not provided immediately, the victim can die. Factors such as wind velocity, amount of humidity, and length of exposure all affect the degree of injury.

Prolonged exposure to the cold can result in **hypothermia,** a condition in which the body temperature is less than 95°F (35°C). Elderly individuals are more susceptible to hypothermia than are younger individuals (figure 16-30). Signs and symptoms include shivering, numbness, weakness or drowsiness, low body temperature, poor coordination, confusion, and loss of consciousness. If prolonged exposure continues, body processes will slow down and death can occur. Treatment consists of getting the victim to a warm area, removing wet clothing, slowly warming the victim by wrapping in blankets or putting on dry clothing, and, if the victim is fully conscious, giving warm nonalcoholic, noncaffeinated liquids by mouth. Avoid warming the victim too quickly, because rapid warming can cause dangerous heart arrhythmias.

Frostbite is actual freezing of tissue fluids accompanied by damage to the skin and underlying tissues (figure 16-31). It is caused by exposure to freezing or below-freezing temperatures.

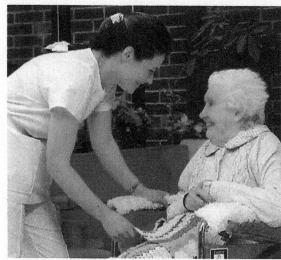

FIGURE 16-30 Elderly individuals are more susceptible to hypothermia than are younger individuals.

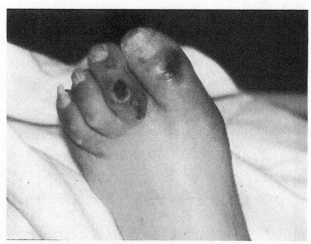

FIGURE 16-31 Frostbite is actual freezing of tissue fluids accompanied by damage to skin and underlying tissues. *(Courtesy of Deborah Funk, MD, Albany Medical Center, Albany, NY)*

Early signs and symptoms include redness and tingling. As frostbite progresses, signs and symptoms include pale, glossy skin, white or grayish yellow in color; blisters; skin that is cold to the touch; numbness; and sometimes, pain that gradually subsides until the victim does not feel any pain. If exposure continues, the victim may become confused, lethargic, and incoherent. Shock may develop followed by unconsciousness and death. First aid for frostbite is directed at maintaining respirations, treating for shock, warming the affected parts, and preventing further injury. Frequently, small areas of the body are affected by frostbite. Common sites include the fingers, toes, ears, nose, and cheeks. Extreme care must be taken to avoid further injury to areas damaged by frostbite. Because the victim usually does not feel pain, the part must be warmed carefully, taking care not to burn the injured tissue. The parts affected may be immersed in warm water at 100–104°F (37.8–40°C).

 CAUTION: Heat lamps, hot water above 104°F (40°C), or heat from a stove or oven should *not* be used. Furthermore, the parts should *not* be rubbed or massaged, because this may cause gangrene (death of the tissue). Avoid opening or breaking any blisters that form because doing so will create an open wound. Do *not* allow the victim to walk or stand if the feet, legs, or toes are affected. Dry, sterile dressings can be placed between toes or fingers to prevent them from rubbing and causing further injury.

Medical help should be obtained as quickly as possible.

Shock is frequently noted in victims exposed to the cold. Be alert for all signs of shock and treat for shock as necessary.

STUDENT: *Go to the workbook and complete the assignment sheet for 16:8, Providing First Aid for Cold Exposure. Then return and continue with the procedure.*

PROCEDURE 16:8

Providing First Aid for Cold Exposure

Equipment and Supplies

Blankets, bath water and thermometer, sterile gauze sponges

Procedure

1. Follow the priorities of care, if indicated:

   a. Check the scene. Move the victim only if absolutely necessary.

   b. Check the victim for consciousness and breathing.

   c. Call emergency medical services (EMS) if necessary.

   d. Provide care to the victim.

   e. Check for bleeding. Control severe bleeding.

   CAUTION: If possible, wear gloves or use a protective barrier while controlling bleeding.

2. Observe the victim closely for signs and symptoms of cold exposure. Information may also be obtained directly from the victim or observers. Note shivering, numbness, weakness or drowsiness, confusion, low body temperature, and lethargy. Check the skin, particularly on the toes, fingers, ears, nose, and cheeks. Suspect frostbite if any areas are pale, glossy, white or grayish yellow, and cold to the touch, and if the victim complains of any part of the body feeling numb or painless.

3. Move the victim to a warm area as soon as possible.

4. Immediately remove any wet or frozen clothing. Loosen any tight clothing that decreases circulation.

5. Slowly warm the victim by wrapping the victim in blankets or dressing the victim in dry, warm clothing. If a body part is affected by frostbite, immerse the part in warm water measuring 100–104°F (37.8–40°C).

   CAUTION: Warm a victim of hypothermia slowly. Rapid warming can cause heart problems or increase circulation to the surface of the body, which causes additional cooling of vital organs.

   CAUTION: Do *not* use heat lamps, hot water above the stated temperatures, or heat from stoves or ovens. Excessive heat can burn the victim.

6. After the body part affected by frostbite has been thawed and the skin becomes flushed, discontinue warming the area because swelling may develop rapidly. Dry the part by blotting gently with a towel or soft cloth. Gently wrap the part in clean or sterile cloths. Use sterile gauze to separate the fingers and/or toes to prevent them from rubbing together.

   CAUTION: *Never* rub or massage the frostbitten area, because doing so can cause gangrene.

7. Help the victim lie down. Do not allow the victim to walk or stand if the legs, feet, or toes are injured. Elevate any injured areas.

PROCEDURE 16:8

8. Observe the victim for signs of shock. Treat for shock as necessary.

9. If the victim is conscious and is not nauseated or vomiting, give warm liquids to drink.

    ▽ **CAUTION:** Do **not** give beverages containing alcohol or caffeine. Give the victim warm broth, water, or milk.

10. Reassure the victim while providing treatment. Remain calm and encourage the victim to remain calm.

11. Obtain medical help as soon as possible.

12. Wash hands thoroughly after providing care.

Practice

Go to the workbook and use the evaluation sheet for 16:8, Providing First Aid for Cold Exposure, to practice this procedure. When you believe you have mastered this skill, sign the sheet and give it to your instructor for further action.

✓ **Final Checkpoint** Using the criteria listed on the evaluation sheet, your instructor will grade your performance.

16:9 INFORMATION

Providing First Aid for Bone and Joint Injuries

Injuries to bones and joints are common in accidents and falls. A variety of injuries can occur to bones and joints. Such injuries sometimes occur together; other times, these injuries occur by themselves. Examples of injuries to bones and joints are fractures, dislocations, sprains, and strains.

FRACTURES

A **fracture** is a break in a bone. A closed, or simple, fracture is a bone break that is not accompanied by an external or open wound on the skin. A compound, or open, fracture is a bone break that is accompanied by an open wound on the skin. The types of fractures are discussed in Chapter 7:4 and shown in figure 7-22.

Signs and symptoms of fractures can vary. Not all signs and symptoms will be present in every victim. Common signs and symptoms include:

♦ deformity

♦ limited motion or loss of motion

♦ pain and tenderness at the fracture site

♦ swelling and discoloration

♦ the protrusion of bone ends through the skin

♦ the victim heard a bone break or snap or felt a grating sensation (crepitation)

♦ abnormal movements within a part of the body

Basic principles of treatment for fractures include:

♦ maintain respirations

♦ treat for shock

♦ keep the broken bone from moving

♦ prevent further injury.

♦ use devices such as splints and slings to prevent movement of the injured part.

♦ obtain medical help whenever a fracture is evident or suspected

DISLOCATIONS

A **dislocation** is when the end of a bone is either displaced from a joint or moved out of its normal position within a joint. This injury is frequently accompanied by a tearing or stretching of ligaments, muscles, and other soft tissue.

Signs and symptoms that may occur include:

♦ deformity

♦ limited or abnormal movement

♦ swelling

♦ discoloration

♦ pain and tenderness

♦ a shortening or lengthening of the affected arm or leg

First aid for dislocations is basically the same as that for fractures. No attempt should be made to reduce the dislocation (that is, replace the bone in the joint). The affected part must be immobilized in the position in which it was found. Immobilization is accomplished by using splints and/or slings. Movement of the injured part can lead to additional injury to nerves, blood vessels, and other tissue in the area. Obtain medical help immediately.

SPRAINS

A **sprain** is an injury to the tissues surrounding a joint; it usually occurs when the part is forced beyond its normal range of movement. Ligaments, tendons, and other tissues are stretched or torn. Common sites for sprains include the ankles and wrists.

Signs and symptoms of a sprain include swelling, pain, discoloration, and sometimes, impaired motion. Frequently, sprains resemble fractures or dislocations. If in doubt, treat the injury as a fracture.

First aid for a sprain includes:

♦ Apply a cold application to decrease swelling and pain

♦ Elevate the affected part

♦ Encourage the victim to rest the affected part

♦ Apply an elastic bandage to provide support for the affected area but avoid stretching the bandage too tightly

♦ Obtain medical help if swelling is severe or if there is any question of a fracture

STRAINS

A **strain** is the overstretching of a muscle; it is caused by overexertion or lifting. A frequent site for strains is the back. Signs and symptoms of a strain include sudden pain, swelling, and/or bruising.

Basic principles of first aid treatment for a strain include:

♦ Encourage the victim to rest the affected muscle while providing support

♦ Recommend bedrest with a backboard under the mattress for a strained back

♦ Apply cold applications to reduce the swelling

♦ After the swelling decreases, apply warm, wet applications because warmth relaxes the muscles; different types of cold and heat packs are available (figure 16-32)

♦ Obtain medical help for severe strains and all back injuries

SPLINTS

Splints are devices that can be used to immobilize injured parts when fractures, dislocations, and other similar injuries are present or suspected. Many commercial splints are available, including inflatable, or air, splints, padded boards, and traction splints. Splints can also be made from cardboard, newspapers, blankets, pillows, boards, and other similar materials. Some basic principles regarding the use of splints are:

♦ Splints should be long enough to immobilize the joint above and below the injured area (figure 16-33). By preventing movement in these joints, the injured bone or area is held in position and further injury is prevented.

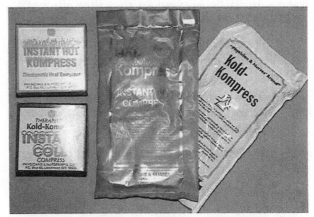

FIGURE 16-32 Disposable heat and cold packs contain chemicals that must be activated before using.

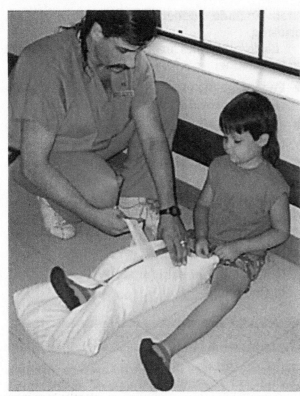

FIGURE 16-33 Splints should be long enough to immobilize the joint above and below the injured area.

♦ Splints should be padded, especially at bony areas and over the site of injury. Cloths, thick dressings, towels, and similar materials can be used as padding.

♦ Strips of cloth, roller gauze, triangular bandages folded into bands or strips, and similar materials can be used to tie splints in place.

♦ Splints must be applied so that they do not put pressure directly over the site of injury.

♦ If an open wound is present, use a sterile dressing to apply pressure and control bleeding.

⊞ **CAUTION:** Wear gloves or use a protective barrier while controlling bleeding to avoid contamination from the blood.

▽ **CAUTION:** Leave the dressing in place, and apply the splint in such a way that it does *not* put pressure on the wound.

♦ *Never* make any attempt to replace broken bones or reduce a fracture or dislocation. Do *not* move the victim. Splint wherever you find the victim.

♦ *Pneumatic* splints are available in various sizes and shapes for different parts of the arms and legs. Care must be taken to avoid any unnecessary movement while the splint is being positioned. There are two main types of pneumatic splints: air (inflatable) and vacuum (deflatable).

If an *air splint* is positioned over a fracture site, air pressure is used to inflate the splint (figure 16-34A). Some air splints have nozzles; these splints are inflated by blowing into the nozzles. Other air splints require the use of pressurized material in cans, while still others are inflated with cool air from a refrigerant solution. The coldness reduces swelling. Care must be taken to avoid overinflating air splints. To test whether the splint is properly inflated, use a thumb to apply slight pressure to the splint; an indentation mark should result.

Vacuum pneumatic splints are deflated after being positioned over a fracture site. Air is removed from the splint with a hand pump or suction pump until the splint molds to the fracture site to provide support (figure 16-34B). Care must be taken to avoid overdeflation of the splint. A pulse site below the splint should be checked to make sure the splint is not applying too much pressure and cutting off circulation.

♦ *Traction splints* are special devices that provide a pulling or traction effect on the injured bone. They are frequently used for fractures of the femur, or thigh bone.

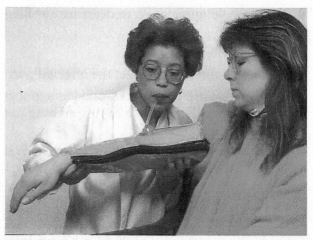

FIGURE 16-34A Some air splints are inflated by blowing into a nozzle. Care must be taken to avoid overinflating this type of splint.

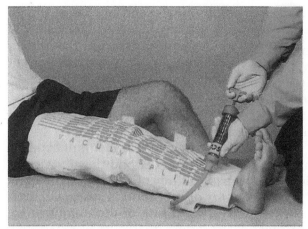

FIGURE 16-34B Vacuum pneumatic splints are deflated until the splint molds to the fracture site to provide support.

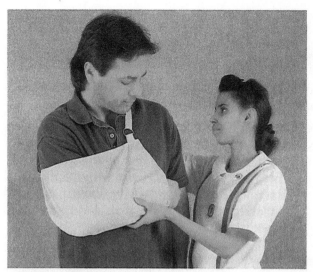

FIGURE 16-35 Commercial slings usually have a series of straps that extend around the neck and/or thoracic region.

CAUTION: Only persons specifically trained in the application of traction splints should apply them.

◆ After a splint is applied, it is essential to note the circulation and the effects on the nerve endings of the skin below the splint to make sure the splint is not too tight. Check skin temperature (it should be warm to the touch), skin color (pale or blue indicates poor circulation), swelling or edema, numbness or tingling, and pulse, if possible.

CAUTION: If any signs of impaired circulation or impaired neurological status are present, immediately loosen the ties holding the splint.

SLINGS

Slings are available in many different forms. Commercial slings usually have a series of straps that extend around the neck and/or thoracic (chest) region (figure 16-35). A common type of sling used for first aid is the triangular bandage. Slings are usually used to support the arm, hand, forearm, and shoulder. They may be used when casts are in place. In addition, they are also used to provide immobility if a fracture of the arm or shoulder is suspected. Basic principles to observe with slings include:

◆ When a sling is applied to an arm, the sling should be positioned in such a way that the hand is higher than the elbow. The purpose of elevating the hand is to promote circulation, prevent swelling (edema), and decrease pain.

◆ Circulation in the limb and nerve supply to the limb must be checked frequently. Specifically, check for skin temperature (should be warm if circulation is good), skin color (blue or very pale indicates poor circulation), swelling (edema), amount of pain, and tingling or numbness. Nail beds can also be used to check circulation. When the nail beds are pressed slightly, they blanch (turn white). If circulation is good, the pink color should return to the nail beds immediately after the pressure is released.

◆ If a sling is being applied because of a suspected fracture to the bone, extreme care must be taken to move the injured limb as little as possible while the sling is being applied. The victim can sometimes help by holding the injured limb in position while the sling is slipped into place.

◆ If a triangular bandage is used, care must be taken so that the knot tied at the neck does not press against a bone. The knot should be tied to either side of the spinal column. Place gauze or padding under the knot of the sling to protect the skin.

◆ When shoulder injuries are suspected, it may be necessary to keep the arm next to the body. After a sling has been applied, another bandage can be placed around the thoracic region to hold the arm against the body.

NECK AND SPINE INJURIES

Injuries to the neck or spine are the most dangerous types of injuries to bones and joints.

 CAUTION: If a victim who has such injuries is moved, permanent damage resulting in paralysis can occur. If at all possible, avoid any movement of a victim with neck or spinal injuries. Wait until a backboard, cervical collar, and adequate help for transfer is available.

SUMMARY

Victims with injuries to bones and/or joints also experience shock. Always be alert for signs of shock and treat as needed.

Injuries to bones and/or joints usually involve a great deal of anxiety, pain, and discomfort, so constantly reassure the victim. Encourage the victim to relax, and position the victim as comfortably as possible. Advise the victim that medical help is on the way. First aid measures are directed toward relieving the pain as much as possible.

Obtain medical help for all victims of bone or joint injuries. The only definite diagnosis of a closed fracture is an X-ray of the area. Whenever a fracture and/or dislocation is suspected, treat the victim as though one of these injuries has occurred.

STUDENT: *Go to the workbook and complete the assignment sheet for 16:9, Providing First Aid for Bone and Joint Injuries. Then return and continue with the procedure.*

PROCEDURE 16:9

Providing First Aid for Bone and Joint Injuries

Equipment and Supplies

Blankets, splints of various sizes, air or inflatable splints, triangular bandages, strips of cloth or roller gauze, disposable gloves

Procedure

1. Follow the priorities of care, if indicated:

   a. Check the scene. Move the victim only if absolutely necessary. If the victim must be moved from a dangerous area, pull in the direction of the long axis of the body (that is, from the head or feet). If at all possible, tie an injured leg to the other leg or secure an injured arm to the body before movement.

    CAUTION: If neck or spinal injuries are suspected, avoid any movement of the victim unless movement is necessary to save the victim's life.

   b. Check the victim for consciousness and breathing.

   c. Call emergency medical services (EMS) if necessary.

   d. Provide care to the victim.

   e. Control severe bleeding. If an open wound accompanies a fracture, take care not to push broken bone ends into the wound.

   CAUTION: If possible, wear gloves or use a protective barrier while controlling bleeding.

2. Observe for signs and symptoms of a fracture, dislocation, or joint injury. Note deformities (such as a shortening or lengthening of an extremity), limited motion or loss of motion, pain, tenderness, swelling, discoloration, and bone

PROCEDURE 16:9

fragments protruding through the skin. Also, the victim may state that he or she heard a bone snap or crack, or may complain of a grating sensation.

3. Immobilize the injured part to prevent movement.

   ▽ **CAUTION:** Do *not* attempt to straighten a deformity, replace broken bone ends, or reduce a dislocation. Avoid any unnecessary movement of the injured part. If a bone injury is suspected, treat the victim as though a fracture or dislocation has occurred. Use splints or slings to immobilize the injury.

4. *To apply splints:*

   a. Obtain commercial splints or improvise splints by using blankets, pillows, newspapers, boards, cardboard, or similar supportive materials.

   b. Make sure that the splints are long enough to immobilize the joint both above and below the injury.

   c. Position the splints, making sure that they do *not* apply pressure directly at the site of injury. Two splints are usually used. However, if a pillow, blanket, or similar item is used, one such item can be rolled around the area to provide support on all sides.

   d. Use thick dressings, cloths, towels, or other similar materials to pad the splints. Make sure bony areas are protected. Avoid direct contact between the splint material and the skin.

   NOTE: Many commercial splints are already padded. However, additional padding is often needed to protect the bony areas.

   e. Use strips of cloth, triangular bandages folded into strips, roller gauze, or other similar material to tie or anchor the splints in place. The use of elastic bandage is discouraged because the bandage may cut off or interfere with circulation. If splints are long, three to five ties may be required. Tie the strips above and below the upper joint and above and below the lower joint. An additional tie should be placed in the center region of the splint.

   f. Avoid any unnecessary movement of the injured area while splints are being applied. If possible, have another individual support the area while you are applying the splints.

5. *To apply air (inflatable) splints:*

   a. Obtain the correct splint for the injured part.

   NOTE: Most air splints are available for full arm, lower arm, wrist, full leg, lower leg, and ankle/foot.

   b. Some air splints have zippers for easier application, but others must be slipped into position on the victim. If the splint has a zipper, position the open splint on the injured area, taking care to avoid any movement of the affected part. Use your hand to support the injured area. Close the zipper. If the splint must be slipped into position, slide the splint onto your arm first. Then hold the injured leg or arm and slide the splint from your arm to the victim's injured extremity. This technique prevents unnecessary movement.

   c. Inflate the splint. Many splints are inflated by blowing into the nozzle. Others require the use of a pressure solution in a can. Follow instructions provided by the manufacturer of the splint.

   d. Check to make sure that the splint is not overinflated. Use your thumb to press a section of the splint. Your thumb should leave a slight indentation if the splint is inflated correctly.

PROCEDURE 16:9

6. *To apply a sling*, follow the manufacturer's instructions for commercial slings. To use a triangular bandage for a sling (figure 16-36), proceed as follows:

   a. If possible, obtain the help of another individual to support the injured arm while the sling is being applied. Sometimes, the victim can hold the injured arm in place.

   b. Place the long straight edge of the triangular bandage on the uninjured side. Allow one end to extend over the shoulder of the uninjured arm. The other end should hang down in front of the victim's chest. The short edge of the triangle should extend back and under the elbow of the injured arm.

   CAUTION: Avoid excessive movement of the injured limb while positioning the sling.

   c. Bring the long end of the bandage up and over the shoulder of the injured arm.

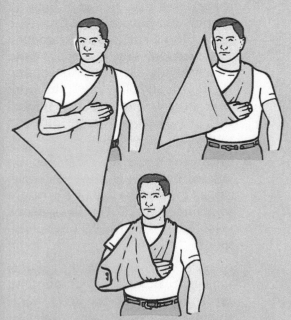

FIGURE 16-36 Steps for applying a triangular bandage as a sling.

   d. Use a square knot to tie the two ends together near the neck. Make sure the knot is not over a bone. Tie it to either side of the spinal column. Place gauze or padding between the knot and the skin. Make sure the hand is elevated 5–6 inches above the elbow.

   e. The point of the bandage is now near the elbow. Bring the point forward, fold it, and pin it to the front of the sling. If no pin is available, coil the end and tie it in a knot.

   CAUTION: If you use a pin, put your hand between the pin and the victim's skin while inserting the pin.

   f. Check the position of the sling. The fingers of the injured hand should extend beyond the edge of the triangular bandage. In addition, the hand should be slightly elevated to prevent swelling (edema).

   g. If a shoulder injury is suspected, it may be necessary to secure the arm close to the body. Apply a large bandage around the thoracic region to stabilize the shoulder joint (figure 16-37).

7. After splints and/or slings have been applied, check for signs of impaired circulation. Skin color should be pink. A

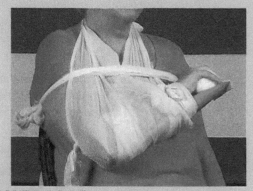

FIGURE 16-37 If a shoulder injury is suspected, use a long bandage to secure the arm against the body to stabilize the shoulder joint.

PROCEDURE 16:9

pale or cyanotic (bluish) color is a sign of poor circulation. The skin should be warm to the touch. Swelling can indicate poor circulation. If the victim complains of pain or pressure from the splints and/or slings, or of numbness or tingling in the area below the splints/sling, circulation may be impaired. Slightly press the nail beds on the foot or hand so they temporarily turn white. If circulation is good, the pink color will return to the nail beds immediately after pressure is released. If you note any signs of impaired circulation, loosen the splints and/or sling immediately.

8. Watch for signs of shock in any victim with a bone and/or joint injury. Remember, inadequate blood flow is the main cause of shock. Watch for signs of impaired circulation, such as a cyanotic (bluish) tinge around the lips or nail beds. Treat for shock, as necessary.

9. If medical help is delayed, cold applications such as cold compresses or an ice bag can be used on the injured area to decrease swelling.

    ▽ **CAUTION:** To prevent injury to the skin, make sure that the ice bag is covered with a towel or other material.

10. Place the victim in a comfortable position, but avoid any unnecessary movement.

▽ **CAUTION:** Avoid *any* movement if a neck or spinal injury is suspected.

11. Reassure the victim while providing first aid. Try to relieve the pain by carefully positioning the injured part, avoiding unnecessary movement, and applying cold.

12. Obtain medical help as quickly as possible.

13. Wash hands thoroughly after providing care.

Practice

Go to the workbook and use the evaluation sheet for 16:9, Providing First Aid for Bone and Joint Injuries, to practice this procedure. When you believe you have mastered this skill, sign the sheet and give it to your instructor for further action.

 Final Checkpoint Using the criteria listed on the evaluation sheet, your instructor will grade your performance.

16:10 INFORMATION

Providing First Aid for Specific Injuries

Although treatment for burns, bleeding, wounds, poisoning, and fractures is basically the same for all regions of the body, injuries to specific body parts require special care. Examples of these parts are the eyes, ears, nose, brain, chest, abdomen, and genital organs.

EYE INJURIES

Any eye injury always involves the danger of vision loss, especially if treated incorrectly. In most cases involving serious injury to the eyes, it is best *not* to provide major treatment. Obtaining medical help, preferably from an eye specialist, is a top priority of first aid care.

♦ *Foreign objects* such as dust, dirt, and similar small particles frequently enter the eye. These objects cause irritation and can scratch the eye or become embedded in the eye tissue. Signs and symptoms include redness, a burning sensation, pain, watering or tearing of the eye, and/or the presence of visible objects in the eye. If the foreign body is floating freely, prevent the victim from rubbing the eye, wash your hands thoroughly, and gently draw the upper lid down over the lower lid. This stimulates the formation of tears. The proximity of the lids also creates a wiping action, which may remove the particle. If this does not remove the foreign body, use your thumb and forefinger to grasp the eyelashes and gently raise the upper eyelid. Tell the victim to look down and tilt his or her head toward the injured side. Use water to gently flush the eye or use the corner of a piece of sterile gauze to gently remove the object.

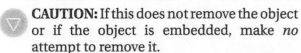

CAUTION: If this does not remove the object or if the object is embedded, make *no* attempt to remove it.

Apply a dry, sterile dressing and obtain medical help for the victim. Serious injury can occur if any attempt is made to remove an object embedded in the eye tissue.

◆ *Blows to the eye* from a fist, accident, or explosion may cause contusions or black eyes as a result of internal bleeding and torn tissues inside the eye. Because this can lead to loss of vision, the victim should be examined as soon as possible by an eye specialist. Apply sterile dressings or an eye shield, keep the victim lying flat, and obtain medical help. It is sometimes best to cover both eyes to prevent involuntary movement of the injured eye.

◆ *Penetrating injuries* that cut the eye tissue are extremely dangerous.

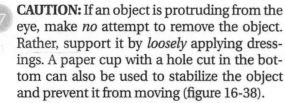

CAUTION: If an object is protruding from the eye, make *no* attempt to remove the object. Rather, support it by *loosely* applying dressings. A paper cup with a hole cut in the bottom can also be used to stabilize the object and prevent it from moving (figure 16-38).

Apply dressings to both eyes to prevent involuntary movement of the injured eye. Avoid applying pressure to the eye while applying the dressings. Keep the victim lying flat on his or her back to prevent fluids from draining out of the eye. Obtain medical help immediately.

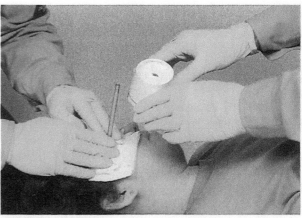

FIGURE 16-38 A cup can be used to stabilize an object impaled in the eye and to prevent it from moving.

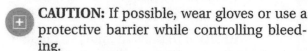

EAR INJURIES

Injuries to the ear can result in rupture or perforation of the eardrum. These injuries also require medical care. Treatment for specific types of ear injuries is as follows:

◆ Wounds of the ear frequently result in torn or detached tissue. Apply sterile dressings with light pressure to control bleeding.

CAUTION: If possible, wear gloves or use a protective barrier while controlling bleeding.

Save any torn tissue and wrap it in gauze moistened with cool sterile water or sterile normal saline solution. Put the gauze wrapped tissue in a plastic bag to keep it cool and moist. Send the torn tissue to the medical facility along with the victim.

NOTE: If sterile water is not available, use cool, clean water.

◆ Keep the victim lying flat, but raise his or her head (if no other conditions prohibit raising the head).

◆ If the eardrum is ruptured or perforated, place sterile gauze loosely in the outer ear canal. Do *not* allow the victim to hit the side of the head in an attempt to restore hearing. Do *not* put any liquids into the ear. Obtain medical help for the victim.

◆ Clear or blood-tinged fluid draining from the ear can be a sign of skull or brain injury. Allow the fluid to flow from the ear. Keep the victim lying down. If possible, turn the victim on his or her injured side and elevate the head and shoulders slightly to allow the fluid to drain. Obtain medical help immediately and report the presence and description of the fluid.

CAUTION: Wear gloves or use a protective barrier to avoid skin contact with fluid draining from the ear.

HEAD OR SKULL INJURIES

Wounds or blows to the head or skull can result in injury to the brain. Again, it is important to obtain medical help as quickly as possible for the victim.

♦ Signs and symptoms of brain injury include clear or blood-tinged cerebrospinal fluid draining from the nose or ears, loss of consciousness, headache, visual disturbances, pupils unequal in size, muscle paralysis, speech disturbances, convulsions, and nausea and vomiting.

♦ Keep the victim lying flat and treat for shock. If there is no evidence of neck or spinal injury, raise the victim's head slightly by supporting the head and shoulders on a small pillow or a rolled blanket or coat.

♦ Watch closely for signs of respiratory distress and provide artificial respiration as needed.

♦ Make *no* attempt to stop the flow of fluid. Loose dressings can be positioned to absorb the flow.

CAUTION: Wear gloves or use a protective barrier to avoid contamination from the cerebrospinal fluid.

♦ Do *not* give the victim any liquids. If the victim complains of excessive thirst, use a clean, cool, wet cloth to moisten the lips, tongue, and inside of the mouth.

♦ If the victim loses consciousness, note how long the victim is unconscious and report this to the emergency rescue personnel.

NOSE INJURIES

Injuries to the nose frequently cause a nosebleed, also called an *epistaxis*. Nosebleeds are usually more frightening than they are serious. Nosebleeds can also be caused by change in altitude, strenuous activity, high blood pressure, and rupture of small blood vessels after a cold. Treatment for a nosebleed includes:

♦ Keep the victim quiet and remain calm.

♦ If possible, place the victim in a sitting position with the head leaning slightly forward.

♦ Apply pressure to control bleeding by pressing the bleeding nostril toward the midline. If both nostrils are bleeding, press both nostrils toward the midline.

   NOTE: If both nostrils are blocked, tell the victim to breathe through the mouth.

CAUTION: Wear gloves or use a protective barrier to avoid contamination from blood.

♦ If application of pressure against the midline or septum does not stop the bleeding, insert a small piece of gauze in the nostril and then apply pressure on the outer surface of the nostril. Be sure to leave a portion of the gauze extending out of the nostril so that the packing can be removed later.

CAUTION: Do not use cotton balls because the fibers will shed and stick.

♦ Apply a cold compress to the bridge of the nose. A covered ice pack or a cold, wet cloth can be used.

♦ If the bleeding does not stop or a fracture of the nose is suspected, obtain medical assistance. If a person has repeated nosebleeds, a referral for medical attention should be made. Nosebleeds can indicate an underlying condition that requires medical care and treatment, such as high blood pressure.

CHEST INJURIES

Injuries to the chest are usually medical emergencies because the heart, lungs, and major blood vessels may be involved. Chest injuries include sucking chest wounds, penetrating wounds, and crushing injuries. In all cases, obtain medical help immediately.

♦ *Sucking chest wound*: This is a deep, open chest wound that allows air to flow directly in and out with breathing. The partial vacuum that is usually present in the pleura (sacs surrounding the lungs) is destroyed, causing the lung on the injured side to collapse. Immediate medical help must be obtained. An airtight dressing must be placed over the wound to prevent air flow into the wound. Aluminum foil, plastic wrap, or other nonporous material should be used to cover the wound. Tape or a bandage can be used to hold the nonporous material in place on three sides. The fourth side should be left loose to allow air to escape when the victim exhales. When the victim inhales, the negative pressure of inspirations will draw the dressing against the wound to create an airtight seal. Maintain an open airway (through the nose or mouth) and provide artificial respiration as needed. If possible, position the victim on his or her injured side and elevate the head and chest slightly. This allows the uninjured lung to expand more freely and prevents pressure on the uninjured lung from blood and damaged tissue.

◆ *Penetrating injuries to the chest*: These injuries can result in sucking chest wounds or damage to the heart and blood vessels. If an object (for example, a knife) is protruding from the chest, do *not* attempt to remove the object. If possible, immobilize the object by placing dressings around it and taping the dressings in position (figure 16-39). Place the victim in a

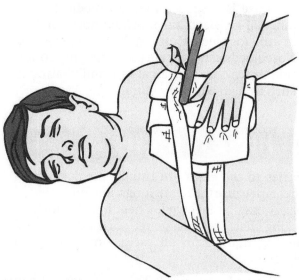

FIGURE 16-39 Immobilize an object protruding from the chest by placing dressings around the object and taping the dressings in place.

comfortable position, maintain respirations, and obtain medical help immediately.

◆ *Crushing chest injuries*: These injuries are caused in vehicular accidents or when heavy objects strike the chest. Fractured ribs and damage to the lungs and/or heart can occur. Place the victim in a comfortable position and, if possible, elevate the head and shoulders to aid breathing. If an injury to the neck or spine is suspected, avoid moving the victim. Obtain medical help immediately.

ABDOMINAL INJURIES

Abdominal injuries can damage internal organs and cause bleeding in major blood vessels. The intestines and other abdominal organs may protrude from an open wound. Medical help must be obtained immediately; bleeding, shock, and organ damage can lead to death in a short period of time.

◆ Signs and symptoms include severe abdominal pain or tenderness, protruding organs, open wounds, nausea and vomiting (particularly of blood), abdominal muscle rigidity, and symptoms of shock.

◆ Position the victim flat on his or her back. Place a pillow or rolled blanket under the knees to bend the knees slightly. This helps relax the abdominal muscles. Elevate the head and shoulders slightly to aid breathing.

◆ Remove clothing from around the wound or protruding organs. Use a large sterile dressing moistened with sterile water or normal saline solution to cover the area. If sterile water or normal saline is not available, use warm tap water to moisten the dressings. Cover the dressings with plastic wrap, if available, to keep the dressings moist. Then cover the dressings with aluminum foil or a folded towel to keep the area warm.

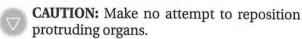 **CAUTION:** Make no attempt to reposition protruding organs.

◆ Avoid giving the victim any fluids or food. If the victim complains of excessive thirst, use a cool, wet cloth to moisten the lips, tongue, and inside of the mouth.

INJURIES TO GENITAL ORGANS

Injuries to genital organs can result from falls, blows, or explosions. Zippers catching on genitals and other accidents sometimes bruise the genitals. Because injuries to the genitals may cause severe pain, bleeding, and shock, medical help is required. Basic principles of first aid include the following:

♦ Control severe bleeding by using a sterile (or clean) dressing to apply direct pressure to the area.

   CAUTION: Wear gloves or use a protective barrier to avoid contamination from blood.

♦ Treat the victim for shock.

♦ Do not remove any penetrating or inserted objects.

♦ Save any torn tissue and wrap it in gauze moistened with cool sterile water or sterile normal saline. Put the gauze-wrapped tissue in a plastic bag to keep it cool and moist. Send the torn tissue to the medical facility along with the victim.

♦ Use a covered ice pack or other cold applications to decrease bleeding and relieve pain.

♦ Obtain medical help.

SUMMARY

Shock frequently occurs in victims with specific injuries to the eyes, ears, chest, abdomen, or other vital organs. Be alert for the signs of shock and immediately treat all victims.

Most of the specific injuries discussed in this section result in extreme pain for the victim. It is essential that you reassure the victim constantly and encourage the victim to relax as much as possible. Direct first aid care toward providing as much relief from pain as possible.

STUDENT: *Go to the workbook and complete the assignment sheet for 16:10, Providing First Aid for Specific Injuries. Then return and continue with the procedure.*

PROCEDURE 16:10

Providing First Aid for Specific Injuries

Equipment and Supplies

Blankets, pillows, dressings, bandages, tape, aluminum foil or plastic wrap, eye shields or sterile dressings, sterile water, disposable gloves

Procedure

1. Follow the priorities of care, if indicated:

   a. Check the scene. Move the victim only if absolutely necessary.

   b. Check the victim for consciousness and breathing.

   c. Call emergency medical services (EMS), if necessary.

   d. Provide care to the victim.

   e. Check for bleeding. Control severe bleeding.

   CAUTION: If possible, wear gloves or use a protective barrier while controlling bleeding.

2. Observe the victim closely for signs and symptoms of specific injuries. Do a systematic examination of the victim. Always have a reason for everything you do. Explain what you are doing to the victim and/or observers.

3. If the victim has an eye injury, proceed as follows:

   a. If the victim has a free-floating particle or foreign body in the eye, warn the victim *not* to rub the eye. Wash your hands thoroughly to prevent infection. Gently grasp the upper eyelid and draw it down over the lower

PROCEDURE 16:10

eyelid. If this does not remove the object, use your thumb and forefinger to grasp the eyelashes and gently raise the upper eyelid. Tell the victim to look down and tilt his or her head slightly to the injured side. Use water to gently flush the eye or use the corner of a piece of sterile gauze to gently remove the object. If this does not remove the object or if the object is embedded, proceed to step b.

b. If an object is embedded in the eye, make *no* attempt to remove it. Rather, apply a dry, sterile dressing to loosely cover the eye. Obtain medical help.

c. If an eye injury has caused a contusion, a black eye, internal bleeding, and/or torn tissue in the eye, apply sterile dressings or eye shields to both eyes. Keep the victim lying flat. Obtain medical help.

NOTE: Both eyes are covered to prevent involuntary movement of the injured eye.

d. If an object is protruding from the eye, make *no* attempt to remove the object. If possible, support the object in position by loosely placing dressings around it. A paper cup with the bottom removed can also be used to surround and prevent any movement of the object. Apply dressings to the uninjured eye to prevent movement of the injured eye. Keep the victim lying flat. Obtain medical help immediately.

4. If the victim has an ear injury:

a. Control severe bleeding from an ear wound by using a sterile dressing to apply light pressure.

CAUTION: Wear gloves or use a protective barrier to prevent contamination from the blood.

b. If any tissue has been torn from the ear, preserve the tissue by placing it in gauze moistened with cool, sterile water or normal saline solution. Place the gauze-wrapped tissue in a plastic bag. Send the torn tissue to the medical facility along with the victim.

NOTE: If sterile water is not available, use cool, clean water.

c. If a rupture or perforation of the eardrum is suspected or evident, place sterile gauze loosely in the outer ear canal. Caution the victim against hitting the side of the head to restore hearing. Obtain medical help.

d. If cerebrospinal fluid is draining from the ear, make no attempt to stop the flow of the fluid. If no neck or spinal injury is suspected, turn the victim on his or her injured side and slightly elevate the head and shoulders to allow the fluid to drain. A dressing may be positioned to absorb the flow. Obtain medical help immediately.

CAUTION: Wear gloves or use a protective barrier to prevent contamination from the cerebrospinal fluid.

5. If the victim has a brain injury:

a. Keep the victim lying flat. Treat for shock. If there is no evidence of a neck or spinal injury, place a small pillow or a rolled blanket or coat under the victim's head and shoulders to elevate the head slightly.

CAUTION: Never position the victim's head lower than the rest of the body.

b. Watch closely for signs of respiratory distress. Provide artificial respiration if needed.

NOTE: Remove the pillow if artificial respiration is given.

c. If cerebrospinal fluid is draining from the ears, nose, and/or mouth, make *no* attempt to stop the flow. Position dressings to absorb the flow.

PROCEDURE 16:10

 CAUTION: Wear gloves or use a protective barrier to prevent contamination from the cerebrospinal fluid.

d. Avoid giving the victim any fluids by mouth. If the victim complains of excessive thirst, use a cool, wet cloth to moisten the lips, tongue, and inside of the mouth.

e. If the victim is unconscious, note for how long and report this information to the emergency rescue personnel.

f. Obtain medical help as quickly as possible.

6. If the victim has a nosebleed:

a. Try to keep the victim calm. Remain calm yourself.

b. Position the victim in a sitting position, if possible. Lean the head forward slightly. If the victim cannot sit up, slightly elevate the head.

c. Apply pressure by pressing the nostril(s) toward the midline. Continue applying pressure for at least 5 minutes and longer if necessary to control the bleeding.

NOTE: If both nostrils are bleeding and must be pressed toward the midline, tell the victim to breathe through the mouth.

 CAUTION: Wear gloves or use a protective barrier to prevent contamination from the blood.

d. If application of pressure does not control the bleeding, insert gauze into the bleeding nostril, taking care to allow some of the gauze to hang out. Then apply pressure again by pushing the nostril toward the midline.

e. Apply cold compresses to the bridge of the nose. Use cold, wet cloths or a covered ice bag.

f. If the bleeding does not stop, a fracture is suspected, or if the victim has repeated nosebleeds, obtain medical help.

NOTE: Nosebleeds can indicate a serious underlying condition that requires medical attention, such as high blood pressure.

7. If the victim has a chest injury:

a. If the wound is a sucking chest wound, apply a nonporous dressing. Use plastic wrap or aluminum foil to create an airtight seal. Use tape on three sides to hold the dressing in place. Leave the fourth side loose to allow excess air to escape when the victim exhales (figure 16-40).

b. Maintain an open airway. Constantly be alert for signs of respiratory distress. Provide artificial respiration as needed.

c. If there is no evidence of a neck or spinal injury, position the victim with his or her injured side down. Slightly elevate the head and chest by placing small pillows or blankets under the victim.

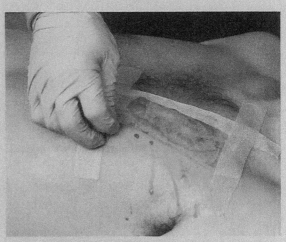

FIGURE 16-40 An airtight dressing is used to cover a sucking chest wound. It is taped on three sides. The fourth side is left open to allow excess air to escape when the victim exhales.

PROCEDURE 16:10

d. If an object is protruding from the chest, make *no* attempt to remove it. If possible, immobilize the object with dressings, and tape around it.

e. Obtain medical help immediately for all chest injuries.

8. If the victim has an abdominal injury:

a. Position the victim flat on the back. Place a small pillow or a rolled blanket or coat under the victim's knees to flex them slightly. Elevate the head and shoulders to aid breathing. If movement of the legs causes pain, leave the victim lying flat.

b. If abdominal organs are protruding from the wound, make *no* attempt to reposition the organs. Remove clothing from around the wound or protruding organs. Use a sterile dressing that has been moistened with sterile water or normal saline solution to cover the area. If sterile water or normal saline is not available, use warm tap water to moisten the dressings.

c. Cover the dressing with plastic wrap, if available, to keep the dressing moist. Then apply a folded towel or aluminum foil to keep the area warm.

d. Avoid giving the victim any fluids or food. If the victim complains of excessive thirst, use a cool, wet cloth to moisten the lips, tongue, and inside of the mouth.

e. Obtain medical help immediately.

9. If the victim has an injury to the genital organs:

a. Control severe bleeding by using a sterile dressing to apply direct pressure.

CAUTION: Wear gloves or use a protective barrier to prevent contamination from the blood.

b. Position the victim flat on the back. Separate the legs to prevent pressure on the genital area.

c. If any tissue is torn from the area, preserve the tissue by wrapping it in gauze moistened with cool, sterile water or normal saline solution. Put the gauze-wrapped tissue in a plastic bag and send it to the medical facility along with the victim.

d. Apply cold compresses such as covered ice bags to the area to relieve pain and reduce swelling.

e. Obtain medical help for the victim.

10. Be alert for the signs of shock in all victims. Treat for shock immediately.

11. Constantly reassure all victims while providing care. Remain calm. Encourage the victim to relax as much as possible.

12. Always obtain medical help as quickly as possible. Shock, pain, and injuries to vital organs can cause death in a very short period of time.

13. Wash hands thoroughly after providing care.

Practice

Go to the workbook and use the evaluation sheet for 16:10, Providing First Aid for Specific Injuries, to practice this procedure. When you believe you have mastered this skill, sign the sheet and give it to your instructor for further action.

Final Checkpoint Using the criteria listed on the evaluation sheet, your instructor will grade your performance.

16:11 INFORMATION

Providing First Aid for Sudden Illness

The victim of a sudden illness requires first aid until medical help can be obtained. Sudden illness can occur in any individual. At times, it is difficult to determine the exact illness being experienced by the victim. However, by knowing the signs and symptoms of some major disorders, you should be able to provide appropriate first aid care. Information regarding a specific condition or illness may also be obtained from the victim, medical alert bracelets or necklaces, or medical information cards. Be alert to all of these factors while caring for the victim of a sudden illness.

HEART ATTACK

A **heart attack** is also called a *coronary thrombosis, coronary occlusion,* or *myocardial infarction*. It may occur when one of the coronary arteries supplying blood to the heart is blocked. If the attack is severe, the victim may die. If the heart stops beating, cardiopulmonary resuscitation (CPR) must be started. Main facts regarding heart attacks are as follows:

♦ Signs and symptoms of a heart attack may vary depending on the amount of heart damage. Severe, painful pressure under the breastbone (sternum) with pain radiating to the shoulders, arms, neck, and jaw is a common symptom (figure 16-41). The victim usually experiences intense shortness of breath. The skin, especially near the lips and nail beds, becomes pale or cyanotic (bluish). The victim feels very weak but is also anxious and apprehensive. Nausea, vomiting, diaphoresis (excessive perspiration), and loss of consciousness may occur.

♦ First aid for a heart attack is directed toward encouraging the victim to relax, placing the victim in a comfortable position to relieve pain and assist breathing, and obtaining medical help. Shock frequently occurs, so provide treatment for shock. Prevent any unnecessary stress and avoid excessive movement because any activity places additional strain on the heart. Reassure the victim constantly, and

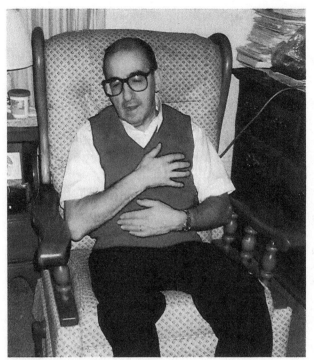

FIGURE 16-41 Severe pressure under the sternum with pain radiating to the shoulders, arms, neck, and jaw is a common symptom of a heart attack.

obtain appropriate medical assistance as soon as possible.

♦ After calling EMS, the American Heart Association recommends that patients who can should take an aspirin. Aspirin keeps platelets in the blood from sticking together to cause a clot. However, there are legal restrictions to which health care providers can administer medications. Only qualified individuals should give the victim aspirin.

CEREBROVASCULAR ACCIDENT OR STROKE

A *stroke* is also called a **cerebrovascular accident** (CVA), *apoplexy,* or *cerebral thrombosis*. It is caused by either the presence of a clot in a cerebral artery that provides blood to the brain or hemorrhage from a blood vessel in the brain.

♦ Signs and symptoms of a stroke vary depending on the part of the brain affected. Some common signs and symptoms are numbness, paralysis, eye pupils unequal in size, mental confusion, slurred speech, nausea, vomiting, difficulty breathing and swallowing, and loss of consciousness.

- First aid for a stroke victim is directed toward maintaining respirations, laying the victim flat on the back with the head slightly elevated or on the side to allow secretions to drain from the mouth, and avoiding any fluids by mouth. Reassure the victim, prevent any unnecessary stress, and avoid any unnecessary movement.

  NOTE: Always remember that although the victim may be unable to speak or may appear to be unconscious, he or she may be able to hear and understand what is going on.

- Obtain medical help as quickly as possible. Immediate care during the first 3 hours can help prevent brain damage. If the CVA is caused by a blood clot, treatment with thrombolytic or "clot busting" drugs such as TPA (tissue plasminogen activator) or angioplasty of the cerebral arteries can dissolve a blood clot and restore blood flow to the brain.

FAINTING

Fainting occurs when there is a temporary reduction in the supply of blood to the brain. It may result in partial or complete loss of consciousness. The victim usually regains consciousness after being in a supine position (that is, lying flat on the back).

- Early signs of fainting include dizziness, extreme pallor, diaphoresis, coldness of the skin, nausea, and a numbness and tingling of the hands and feet.

- If early symptoms are noted, help the victim to lie down or to sit in a chair and position his or her head at the level of the knees.

- If the victim loses consciousness, try to prevent injury. Provide first aid by keeping the victim in a supine position. If no neck or spine injuries are suspected, use a pillow or blankets to elevate the victim's legs and feet 12 inches. Loosen any tight clothing and maintain an open airway. Use cool water to gently bathe the victim's face. Check for any injuries that may have been caused by the fall. Permit the victim to remain flat and quiet until color improves and the victim has recovered. Then

allow the victim to get up gradually. If recovery is not prompt, if other injuries occur or are suspected, or if fainting occurs again, obtain medical help. Fainting can be a sign of a serious illness or condition that requires medical attention.

CONVULSION

A **convulsion,** which is a type of *seizure*, is a strong, involuntary contraction of muscles. Convulsions may occur in conjunction with high body temperatures, head injuries, brain disease, and brain disorders such as epilepsy.

- Convulsions cause a rigidity of body muscles followed by jerking movements. During a convulsion, a person may stop breathing, bite the tongue, lose bladder and bowel control, and injure body parts. The face and lips may develop a cyanotic (bluish) color. The victim may lose consciousness. After regaining consciousness at the end of the convulsion, the victim may be confused and disoriented, and complain of a headache.

- First aid is directed toward preventing self-injury. Removing dangerous objects from the area, providing a pillow or cushion under the victim's head, and providing artificial respiration, as necessary, are all ways to assist the victim.

- Do *not* try to place anything between the victim's teeth. This can cause severe injury to your fingers, and/or damage to the victim's teeth or gums.

- Do *not* use force to restrain or stop the muscle movements; this only causes the contractions to become more severe.

- When the convulsion is over, watch the victim closely. If fluid, such as saliva or vomit, is in the victim's mouth, position the victim on his or her side to allow the fluid to drain from the mouth. Allow the victim to sleep or rest.

- Obtain medical help if the seizure lasts more than a few minutes, if the victim has repeated seizures, if other severe injuries are apparent, if the victim does not have a history of seizures, or if the victim does not regain consciousness.

DIABETIC REACTIONS

Diabetes mellitus is a metabolic disorder caused by a lack or insufficient production of insulin (a hormone produced by the pancreas). Insulin helps the body transport glucose, a form of sugar, from the bloodstream into body cells where the glucose is used to produce energy. When there is a lack of insulin, sugar builds up in the bloodstream. Insulin injections can reduce and control the level of sugar in the blood. Individuals with diabetes are in danger of developing two condi-

tions that require first aid: diabetic coma and insulin shock (figure 16-42).

◆ **Diabetic coma** or *hyperglycemia* is caused by an increase in the level of glucose in the bloodstream. The condition may result from an excess intake of sugar, failure to take insulin, or insufficient production of insulin. Signs and symptoms include confusion; weakness or dizziness; nausea and/or vomiting; rapid, deep respirations; dry, flushed skin; and a sweet or fruity odor to the breath. The victim will eventually lose consciousness and die unless the

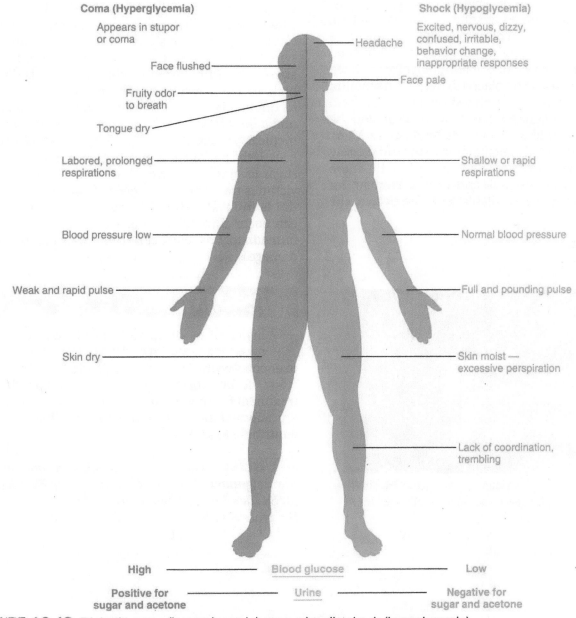

FIGURE 16-42 Diabetic coma (hyperglycemia) versus insulin shock (hypoglycemia).

condition is treated. Medical assistance must be obtained as quickly as possible.

♦ **Insulin shock** or *hypoglycemia* is caused by an excess amount of insulin (and a low level of glucose) in the bloodstream. It may result from failure to eat the recommended amounts, vomiting after taking insulin, or taking excessive amounts of insulin. Signs and symptoms include muscle weakness; mental confusion; restlessness or anxiety; diaphoresis; pale, moist skin; hunger pangs; and/or palpitations (rapid, irregular heartbeats). The victim may lapse into a coma and develop convulsions. The onset of insulin shock is sudden, and the victim's condition can deteriorate quickly; therefore, immediate first aid care is required. If the victim is conscious, give him or her a drink containing sugar, such as sweetened orange juice. A cube or teaspoon of granulated sugar can also be placed in the victim's mouth. If the victim is confused, avoid giving hard candy. Unconsciousness could occur, and the victim could choke on the hard candy. Many individuals with diabetes use tubes of glucose that they carry with them (figure 16-43). If the victim is conscious and can swallow and a glucose tube is available, it can be given to the victim.

The intake of sugar should quickly control the reaction. If the victim loses consciousness or convulsions start, provide care for the convulsions and obtain medical assistance immediately.

By observing symptoms carefully and obtaining as much information as possible from the victim, you can usually determine whether the condition is diabetic coma or insulin shock. Ask the victim, "Have you eaten today?" and "Have you taken your insulin?" If the victim has taken insulin but has not eaten, insulin shock is developing because there is too much insulin in the body. If the victim has eaten but has not taken insulin, diabetic coma is developing. In cases when you know that the victim is diabetic but the victim is unconscious and there are no definite symptoms of either condition, you may not be able to determine whether the condition is diabetic coma or insulin shock. In such cases, the recommendation is to put granulated sugar under the victim's tongue and activate emergency medical services (EMS). This is the lesser of two evils. If the patient is in diabetic coma, the blood-sugar level can be lowered as needed when the victim is transported for medical care. If the victim is in insulin shock, however, brain damage can occur if the blood-sugar level is not raised immediately. Medical care cannot correct brain damage.

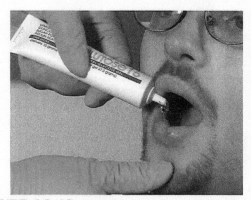

FIGURE 16-43 A victim experiencing insulin shock needs glucose or some form of sugar as quickly as possible.

SUMMARY

In all cases of sudden illness, constantly reassure the victim and make every attempt to encourage the victim to relax and avoid further stress. Be alert for the signs of shock and provide treatment for shock to all victims. The pain, anxiety, and fear associated with sudden illness can contribute to shock.

STUDENT: *Go to the workbook and complete the assignment sheet for 16:11, Providing First Aid for Sudden Illness. Then return and continue with the procedure.*

PROCEDURE 16:11

Providing First Aid for Sudden Illness

Equipment and Supplies

Blankets, pillows, sugar, clean cloth, cool water, disposable gloves

Procedure

1. Follow the priorities of care, if indicated.

   a. Check the scene. Move the victim only if absolutely necessary.

   b. Check the victim for consciousness and breathing.

   c. Call emergency medical services (EMS), if necessary.

   d. Provide care to the victim.

   e. Check for bleeding. Control severe bleeding.

   CAUTION: If possible, wear gloves or use a protective barrier while controlling bleeding.

2. Closely observe the victim for specific signs and symptoms. If the victim is conscious, obtain information about the history of the illness, type and amount of pain, and other pertinent details. If the victim is unconscious, check for a medical bracelet or necklace or a medical information card. Always have a reason for everything you do. Explain your actions to any observers, especially if it is necessary to check the victim's wallet for a medical card.

3. If you suspect the victim is having a *heart attack*, provide first aid as follows:

   a. Place the victim in the most comfortable position possible, but avoid unnecessary movement. Some victims will want to lie flat, but others will want to be in a partial or complete sitting position. If the victim is having difficulty breathing, use pillows or rolled blankets to elevate the head and shoulders.

   b. Obtain medical help for the victim immediately. Advise EMS that oxygen may be necessary.

   c. Encourage the victim to relax. Reassure the victim. Remain calm and encourage others to remain calm.

   d. Watch for signs of shock and treat for shock as necessary. Avoid overheating the victim.

   e. If the victim complains of excessive thirst, use a wet cloth to moisten the lips, tongue, and inside of the mouth. Small sips of water can also be given to the victim, but avoid giving large amounts of fluid.

   CAUTION: Do *not* give the victim ice water or very cold water because the cold can intensify shock.

4. If you suspect that the victim has had a *stroke*:

   a. Place the victim in a comfortable position. Keep the victim lying flat or slightly elevate the victim's head and shoulders to aid breathing. If the victim has difficulty swallowing, turn the victim on his or her side to allow secretions to drain from the mouth and prevent choking on the secretions.

   b. Reassure the victim. Encourage the victim to relax.

   c. Avoid giving the victim any fluids or food by mouth. If the victim complains of excessive thirst, use a cool, wet cloth to moisten the lips, tongue, and inside of the mouth.

   d. Obtain medical help for the victim as quickly as possible.

PROCEDURE 16:11

5. If the victim has *fainted*:

   a. Keep the victim in a supine position (that is, lying flat on the back). Raise the legs and feet 12 inches.

   b. Check for breathing. Provide artificial respiration, if necessary.

   c. Loosen any tight clothing.

   d. Use cool water to gently bathe the face.

   e. Check for any other injuries.

   f. Encourage the victim to continue lying down until his or her skin color improves.

   g. If no other injuries are suspected, allow the victim to get up slowly. First, elevate the head and shoulders. Then place the victim in a sitting position. Allow the victim to stand slowly. If any signs of dizziness, weakness, or pallor are noted, return the victim to the supine position.

   h. If the victim does not recover quickly, or if any other injuries occur, obtain medical care. If fainting has occurred frequently, refer the victim for medical care.

   NOTE: Fainting can be a sign of a serious illness or condition.

6. If the victim is having a *convulsion*:

   a. Remove any dangerous objects from the area. If the victim is near heavy furniture or machinery that cannot be moved, move the victim to a safe area.

   b. Place soft material such as a blanket, small pillow, rolled jacket, or other similar material under the victim's head to prevent injury.

   c. Closely observe respirations at all times. During the convulsion, there will be short periods of apnea (cessation of breathing).

NOTE: If breathing does not resume quickly, artificial respiration may be necessary.

   d. Do *not* try to place anything between the victim's teeth. This can cause injury to the teeth and/or gums.

   e. Do *not* attempt to restrain the muscle contractions. This only makes the contractions more severe.

   f. Note how long the convulsion lasts and what parts of the body are involved. Be sure to report this information to the EMS personnel.

   g. After the convulsion ends, closely watch the victim. Encourage the victim to rest.

   h. Obtain medical assistance if the convulsion lasts more than a few minutes, if the victim has repeated convulsions, if other severe injuries are apparent, if the victim does not have a history of convulsions, or if the victim does not regain consciousness.

7. If the victim is in *diabetic coma*:

   a. Place the victim in a comfortable position. If the victim is unconscious, position him or her on either side to allow secretions to drain from the mouth.

   b. Frequently check respirations. Provide artificial respiration as needed.

   c. Obtain medical help immediately so the victim can be transported to a medical facility.

8. If the victim is in *insulin shock*:

   a. If the victim is conscious and can swallow, offer a drink containing sugar or oral glucose if a tube is available.

   b. If the victim is unconscious, place a small amount of granulated sugar under the victim's tongue.

PROCEDURE 16:11

c. Place the victim in a comfortable position. Position an unconscious victim on either side to allow secretions to drain from the mouth.

d. If recovery is not prompt, obtain medical help immediately.

9. Observe all victims of sudden illness for signs of shock. Treat for shock as necessary.

10. Constantly reassure any victim of sudden illness. Encourage relaxation to decrease stress.

11. Wash hands thoroughly after providing care.

Practice

Go to the workbook and use the evaluation sheet for 16:11, Providing First Aid for Sudden Illness, to practice this procedure. When you believe you have mastered this skill, sign the sheet and give it to your instructor for further action.

✔ **Final Checkpoint** Using the criteria listed on the evaluation sheet, your instructor will grade your performance.

16:12 INFORMATION

Applying Dressings and Bandages

In many cases requiring first aid, it will be necessary for you to apply dressings and bandages. This section provides basic information on types of bandages and dressings and on application methods.

A **dressing** is a sterile covering placed over a wound or an injured part. It is used to control bleeding, absorb blood and secretions, prevent infection, and ease pain. Materials that may be used as dressings include gauze pads in a variety of sizes and compresses of thick, absorbent material (figure 16-44). Fluff cotton should *not* be used as a dressing because the loose cotton fibers may contaminate the wound. In an emergency when no dressings are available, a clean handkerchief or pillowcase may be used. The dressing is held in place with tape or a bandage.

Bandages are materials used to hold dressings in place, to secure splints, and to support and protect body parts. Bandages should be applied snugly enough to control bleeding and prevent movement of the dressing, but not so tightly that they interfere with circulation. Types of bandages include roller gauze bandages, triangular bandages, and elastic bandages (figure 16-45).

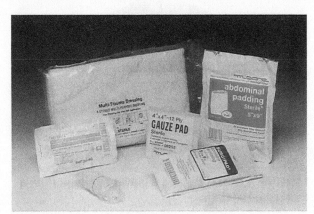

FIGURE 16-44 Dressings to cover a wound are available in many different sizes.

◆ *Roller gauze bandages* come in a variety of widths, most commonly 1-, 2-, and 3-inch widths. They can be used to hold dressings in place on almost any part of the body.

◆ *Triangular bandages* can be used to secure dressings on the head/scalp or as slings. A triangular bandage is sometimes used as a covering for a large body part such as a hand, foot, or shoulder. By folding the triangular bandage into a band of cloth called a *cravat* (figure 16-46), the bandage can be used to secure splints or dressings on body parts.

◆ *Elastic bandages* are easy to apply because they readily conform, or mold, to the injured

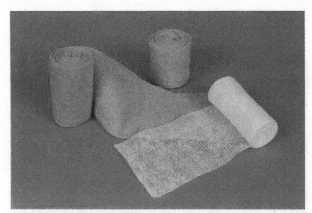

FIGURE 16-45 Roller gauze and elastic bandages can be used to hold dressings in place.

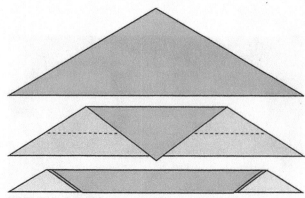

FIGURE 16-46 Folding a cravat bandage from a triangular bandage.

part. However, they can be quite hazardous; if they are applied too tightly or are stretched during application, they can cut off or constrict circulation. Elastic bandages are sometimes used to provide support and stimulate circulation.

Several methods are used to wrap bandages. The method used depends on the body part involved. Some common wraps include the spiral wrap, the figure-eight wrap for joints, and the finger, or recurrent, wrap. The wraps are described in Procedure 16:12, immediately following this information section.

After any bandage has been applied, it is important to check the body part below the bandage to make sure the bandage is not so tight as to interfere with blood circulation. Signs that indicate poor circulation include swelling, a pale or blue (cyanotic) color to the skin, coldness to the touch, and numbness or tingling. If the bandage has been applied to the hand, arm, leg, or foot, press lightly on the nail beds to blanch them (that is, make them turn white). The pink color should return to the nail beds immediately after pressure is released. If the pink color does not return or returns slowly, this is an indication of poor or impaired circulation. If any signs of impaired circulation are noted, loosen the bandages immediately.

STUDENT: *Go to the workbook and complete the assignment sheet for 16:12, Applying Dressings and Bandages. Then return and continue with the procedure.*

PROCEDURE 16:12

Applying Dressings and Bandages

Equipment and Supplies

Sterile gauze pads, triangular bandage, roller gauze bandage, elastic bandage, tape, disposable gloves

Procedure

1. Assemble equipment.

2. Wash hands. Put on gloves if there is any chance of contact with blood or body fluids.

3. Apply a dressing to a wound as follows:

   a. Obtain the correct size dressing. The dressing should be large enough to extend at least 1 inch beyond the edges of the wound.

   b. Open the sterile dressing package, taking care not to touch or handle the sterile dressing with your fingers.

PROCEDURE 16:12

c. Use a pinching action to pick up the sterile dressing so you handle only one part of the outside of the dressing. The ideal situation would involve the use of sterile transfer forceps or sterile gloves to handle the dressing. However, these items are usually not available in emergency situations.

d. Place the dressing on the wound. The untouched (sterile) side of the dressing should be placed on the wound. Do *not* slide the dressing into position. Instead, hold the dressing directly over the wound and then lower the dressing onto the wound.

e. Secure the dressing in place with tape or with one of the bandage wraps.

▽ **CAUTION:** If tape is used, do not wrap it completely around the part. This can lead to impaired circulation.

4. Apply a triangular bandage to the head or scalp (figure 16-47):

a. Fold a 2-inch hem on the base (longest side) of the triangular bandage.

b. Position and secure a sterile dressing in place over the wound.

c. Keeping the hem on the outside, position the middle of the base of the bandage on the forehead, just above the eyebrows.

d. Bring the point of the bandage down over the back of the head.

e. Bring the two ends of the base of the bandage around the head and above the ears. Cross the ends when they meet at the back of the head. Bring them around to the forehead.

f. Use a square knot to tie the ends in the center of the forehead.

g. Use one hand to support the head. Use the other hand to gently but firmly pull down on the point of the bandage at the back of the head until

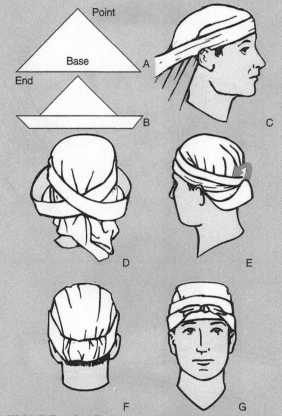

FIGURE 16-47 Steps for applying a triangular bandage to the head or scalp.

the bandage is snug against the head.

h. Bring the point up and tuck it into the bandage where the bandage crosses at the back of the head.

5. Make a cravat bandage from a triangular bandage (review figure 16-46):

a. Bring the point of the triangular bandage down to the middle of the base (the long end of the bandage).

b. Continue folding the bandage lengthwise until the desired width is obtained.

6. Apply a circular bandage with the cravat bandage (figure 16-48):

a. Place a sterile dressing on the wound.

PROCEDURE 16:12

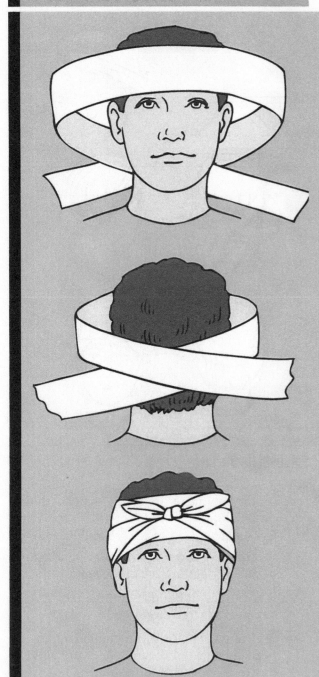

FIGURE 16-48 Steps for applying a circular bandage with a cravat bandage.

b. Place the center of the cravat bandage over the sterile dressing.

c. Bring the ends of the cravat around the body part and cross them when they meet.

d. Bring the ends back to the starting point.

e. Use a square knot to tie the ends of the cravat over the dressing.

▽ **CAUTION:** Avoid tying or wrapping the bandage too tightly. This could impair circulation.

NOTE: Roller gauze bandage can also be used.

▽ **CAUTION:** This type of wrap is *never* used around the neck because it could strangle the victim.

7. Apply a spiral wrap using roller gauze bandage or elastic bandage:

a. Place a sterile dressing over the wound.

b. Hold the roller gauze or elastic bandage so that the loose end is hanging off the bottom of the roll.

c. Start at the farthest end (the bottom of the limb) and move in an upward direction.

d. Anchor the bandage by placing it on an angle at the starting point. To do this, encircle the limb once, leaving a corner of the bandage uncovered. Turn down this free corner and then encircle the part again with the bandage (figure 16-49A).

e. Continue encircling the limb. Use a spiral type motion to move up the limb. Overlap each new turn approximately half the width of the bandage.

f. Use one or two circular turns to finish the wrap at the end point.

PROCEDURE 16:12

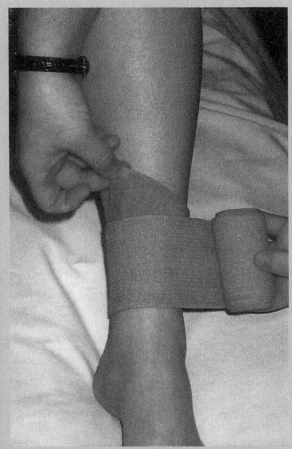

FIGURE 16-49A Anchor the bandage by leaving a corner exposed. This corner is then folded down and covered when the bandage is circled around the limb.

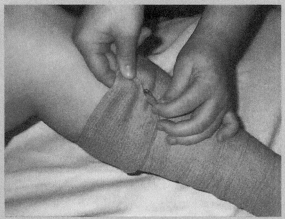

FIGURE 16-49B Place your hand between the bandage and the victim's skin while inserting a pin.

c. Make one or two circular turns around the instep and foot (figure 16-50A).

d. Bring the bandage up over the foot in a diagonal direction. Bring it around the back of the ankle and then down over the top of the foot. Circle it under the instep. This creates the figure-eight pattern.

e. Repeat the figure-eight pattern. With each successive turn, move downward and backward toward the heel

g. Secure the end by taping, pinning, or tying. To avoid injury when pins are used, place your hand under the double layer of bandage and between the pin and the skin before inserting the pin (figure 16-49B). The end of the bandage can also be cut in half and the two halves brought around opposite sides and tied into place.

8. Use roller gauze bandage or elastic bandage to apply a figure-eight ankle wrap:

a. Position a dressing over the wound.

b. Anchor the bandage at the instep of the foot.

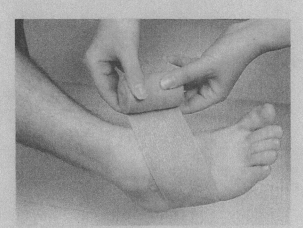

FIGURE 16-50A Bring the bandage over the foot in a diagonal direction for the start of the figure-eight pattern.

PROCEDURE 16:12

(figure 16-50B). Overlap the previous turn by one-half to two-thirds the width of the bandage.

NOTE: Hold the bandage firmly but do not pull it too tightly. If you are using elastic bandage, avoid stretching the material during the application.

f. Near completion, use one or two final circular wraps to circle the ankle.

g. Secure the bandage in place by taping, pinning, or tying the ends, as described in step 7g.

▽ **CAUTION:** To avoid injury to the victim when pins are used, place your hand between the bandage and the victim's skin.

9. Use roller gauze bandage to apply a recurrent wrap to the fingers (figure 16-51).

a. Place a sterile dressing over the wound.

b. Hold the roller gauze bandage so that the loose end is hanging off the bottom of the roll.

c. Place the end of the bandage on the bottom of the finger. Then bring the bandage up to the tip of the finger and down to the bottom of the oppo-

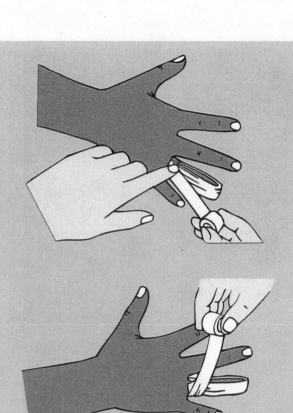

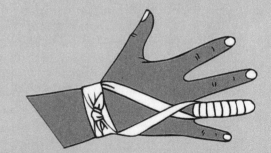

FIGURE 16-51 Recurrent wrap for the finger

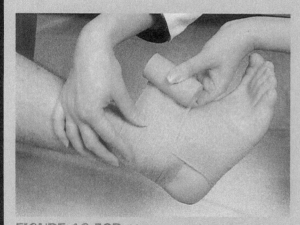

FIGURE 16-50B Keep repeating the figure-eight pattern by moving downward and backward toward the heel with each turn.

PROCEDURE 16:12

site side of the finger. With overlapping wraps, fold the bandage backward and forward over the finger three or four times.

d. Start at the bottom of the finger and use a spiral wrap up and down the finger to hold the recurrent wraps in position.

e. Complete the bandage by using a figure-eight wrap around the wrist. Bring the bandage in a diagonal direction across the back of the hand. Circle the wrist at least two times. Bring the bandage back over the top of the hand and circle the bandaged finger. Repeat this figure-eight motion at least twice.

f. Secure the bandage by circling the wrist once or twice. Tie the bandage at the wrist.

10. After any bandage has been applied, check the circulation below the bandage at frequent intervals. If possible, check for a pulse at a site below the bandage. Note any signs of impaired circulation, including swelling, coldness, numbness or tingling, pallor or cyanosis, and poor return of pink color after nail beds are blanched by lightly pressing on them. If any signs of poor circulation are noted, loosen the bandages immediately.

11. Obtain medical help for any victim who may need additional care.

12. Remove gloves and wash hands.

Practice

Go to the workbook and use the evaluation sheet for 16:12, Applying Dressings and Bandages, to practice this procedure. When you believe you have mastered this skill, sign the sheet and give it to your instructor for further action.

 Final Checkpoint Using the criteria listed on the evaluation sheet, your instructor will grade your performance.

CHAPTER 16 SUMMARY

First aid is defined as "the immediate care given to the victim of an injury or illness to minimize the effect of the injury or illness until experts can take over." Nearly everyone at some time experiences situations for which a proper knowledge of first aid is essential. It is important to follow correct techniques while administering first aid and to provide only the treatment you are qualified to provide.

The basic principles of first aid were presented in this unit. Methods of cardiopulmonary resuscitation (CPR) for infants, children, adults, and choking victims were described. Proper first aid for bleeding, shock, poisoning, burns, heat and cold exposure, bone and joint injuries, specific injuries, and sudden illness were covered. Instructions were given for the application of common dressings and bandages. By learning and following the suggested methods, the health care worker can provide correct first aid treatment in emergency situations until the help of experts can be obtained.

TODAY'S RESEARCH: TOMORROW'S HEALTH CARE

A microchip to cure diabetes?

Diabetes mellitus is a chronic disease caused by a decreased secretion of insulin, a hormone that is needed by body cells to absorb glucose (sugar) from the blood. In the United States, approximately 18.2 million people, or 6.3 percent of the population, have diabetes. Many of these individuals have insulin-dependent diabetes, which means they must inject daily doses of insulin to maintain blood glucose levels. For years, researchers have been looking for a technology that will end the need for individuals with diabetes to use needles to inject insulin and to constantly prick the skin to draw blood for glucose monitoring.

One researcher, Tejal Desai, has been successful in curing rats with diabetes by using a biological microelectromechanical system (MEMS), commonly called bioMEMS. BioMEMS are tiny devices that use microchips. Desai built a small implantable capsule with tiny pores, smaller than 1/100 of a human hair, on the surface. She placed live insulin-secreting pancreatic cells inside the capsule. The tiny pores on the capsule allow nutrients, waste products, and insulin to pass through, but are so small they prohibit harmful antibodies from entering the capsule. Because the body does not like foreign objects in the bloodstream, it produces antibodies to kill the objects. By blocking the antibodies, Desai appears to have eliminated the problem of rejection, allowing the implanted device to remain in the body where it can monitor the blood glucose level and secrete insulin as needed.

It will be several more years before Desai's research will be used on humans, but many scientists are currently using her ideas to create bioMEMS that can be used to cure disease. Some researchers are evaluating capsules that secrete blood-clotting factors for individuals with hemophilia. Others are trying to develop capsules that will carry dopamine to treat Parkinson's disease. Think of a future in which tiny capsules floating in the bloodstream or implanted in the body cure chronic diseases and allow individuals to live long and healthy lives.

INTERNET SEARCHES

Use the suggested search engines in Chapter 12:4 of this textbook to search the Internet for additional information on the following topics:

1. *Organizations*: find Web sites for the American Red Cross, the American Heart Association, Emergency Medical Services, and Poison Control Centers to learn services offered

2. *CPR*: look for sites that discuss the principles of cardiopulmonary resuscitation, abdominal thrusts, and cardiac emergencies

3. *Automated external defibrillators*: search for manufacturers of AEDs and compare different models

4. *First aid treatments*: find information on recommended treatment for bleeding, wounds, shock, poisoning, snakebites, insect stings, ticks, burns, heat exposure, heat stroke, hypothermia, frostbite, fractures, dislocations, sprains, strains, eye injuries, nose injuries, head and skull injuries, spine injuries, chest injuries, abdominal injuries, myocardial infarction, cerebrovascular accident, fainting, convulsions or seizures, diabetic coma, and insulin shock

REVIEW QUESTIONS

Review the following case histories. List the correct first aid care, in proper order of use, that should be used to treat each victim.

1. You are slicing carrots and cut off the end of your finger.

2. You find your 2-year-old brother in the bathroom. An empty bottle of aspirin tablets is on the floor. His mouth is covered with a white powdery residue.

3. You are watching television with your parents. Suddenly your father complains of severe pain in his chest and left arm. He is very short of breath and his lips appear cyanotic.

4. You are working in chemistry lab. Suddenly an experiment boils over and concentrated hydrochloric acid splashes into your lab partner's face and eyes. She starts screaming with pain.

5. You are driving and the car ahead of you loses control, goes off the road, and hits a tree. When you get to the car, the driver is slumped over the wheel. His arm is twisted at an odd angle. You notice a small fire at the rear of the car. A small child is crying in a car seat in the back seat.

6. You are playing tennis on a hot summer day with a friend. Suddenly your friend collapses on the tennis court. When you get to her, her skin is hot, red, and dry. She is breathing but she is unconscious.

For additional information on first aid and emergency care, write to:

♦ American Red Cross—contact your local chapter for First Aid and CPR courses and certification, or check the Web site at: *www.redcross.org*

♦ American Heart Association—contact your local chapter for CPR courses and certification or check the Web site at: *www.americanheart.org*

♦ Contact the National Highway Traffic Safety Administration (NHTSA), U.S. Department of Transportation, Emergency Medical Services Branch N-42-13, Washington, D.C. 20540 or check the Web at: *www.nhtsa.dot.gov* (click link to traffic safety and then emergency medical services)